The
Corner
Drugstore

The Corner Drugstore

MAX LEBER, R.Ph., B.S.

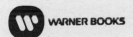
WARNER BOOKS

A Warner Communications Company

The appendix was originally published as *Drug Awareness*
by the Author and Mark Rathgeber.
Copyright © 1977, 1979 by Max R. Leber and Mark Rathgeber

Copyright © 1983 by Max Leber

Warner Books, Inc., 75 Rockefeller Plaza, New York, N.Y. 10019

W A Warner Communications Company

Printed in the United States of America

First printing: January 1983
10 9 8 7 6 5 4 3 2 1

Designed by Giorgetta Bell McRee

Library of Congress Cataloging in Publication Data

Leber, Max.
The corner drugstore.

Includes index.
1. Drugs, Nonprescription.   2. Toilet preparations.
3. Medicine, Popular. I. Title.
RM671.A1L4   615'.1   82-7015
ISBN 0-446-97989-9 (U.S.A.)   AACR2
ISBN 0-446-37278-1 (Canada)

I would like to dedicate this book to all pharmacists, men and women, no matter what area of pharmacy they're in, for all the time and dedication they put into helping people understand more about the medicines that doctors prescribe for them and for helping people make the selection of the over-the-counter medicine that will do the best job for them. In doing this they are creating an image for the pharmacist as a true professional and a vital source of health information in the community.

I would especially like to dedicate the book to Medicine Shoppe International and to the pharmacists associated with it. Medicine Shoppe International is a nationwide chain of independently owned pharmacies that are constantly working to keep the image of the neighborhood pharmacy alive and well. By getting actively involved in their communities, they bring to pharmacy the type of recognition that it so rightly deserves as an important part of the health-care system.

CONTENTS

ACKNOWLEDGMENTS

CONNIE SCHULTE

I would like to thank Connie for all the hours and time over and above her normal working hours in which she typed out the manuscript from my handwritten copies. Now Connie knows what it's like to be a pharmacist and read a doctor's writing.

LINDA AMES

The work Linda put into retyping the corrected manuscript was terrific. Linda, aside from working a full day, had to take care of her small children. How she found the time to type the finished manuscript in perfect form is something I haven't figured out.

DENISE ANGLIN

Denise has been a loyal and dedicated employee of mine for eleven years. She also has the eye of an eagle, because she helped proofread the finished book and caught mistakes that even I didn't see.

JOSEPH CRABTREE

I want to thank Joe Crabtree of J. C. Photographics for spending an evening taking excellent photographs of me for the back cover of the book.

INTRODUCTION

For many people the old Corner Drugstore was part of growing up. It actually was more than just an ordinary drugstore, it was a gathering place for people in the neighborhood. While teenagers were discussing Saturday night's dates, others were catching up on the latest gossip and starting new rumors. Oh yes, the Corner Drugstore is as American as apple pie.

Many of us considered it a valuable source of information about how to treat various common ills and ailments. We relied on our pharmacist for information about all types of over-the-counter medicines, as well as prescription drugs. If we just weren't feeling well, we knew we could go to the Corner Drugstore and leave it to the pharmacist to recommend the right product or the right treatment. An important feature of the Corner Drugstore was that you had to ask the pharmacist for over-the-counter medicines, and he would usually take that product off a shelf behind the counter. I realize that this may not seem important, but it was. For if you had any questions, you could ask them directly of the pharmacist at the time you bought the product.

Then, too, there was an atmosphere in the Corner Drugstore that will never be duplicated. I began working at my neighborhood drugstore, across the street from my house, when I was in high school. The job was just sweeping the floor and stocking the shelves. But it was the place where I decided that I wanted to become a pharmacist. Every day after school, when I worked at the Corner Drugstore, I was intrigued by watching the pharmacist help the people who came in, and by how he seemed to be a friendly part of each family. But the old Corner Drugstore where I began working is today a restaurant. What happened to that Corner Drugstore is what happened to Corner Drugstores everywhere. They are becoming a thing of the past; nowadays we have the large, self-service discount drugstores. As a matter of fact, you can hardly pass a shopping center, or even go into a grocery store, without finding medicine or drugs. The new self-service drugstores certainly offer a larger variety of products to choose from, and the prices are a little cheaper, compared to the Corner Drugstore's. But the self-service stores also allow you to become your own doctor. When you see something advertised on television, or read about a certain product in a magazine, there is nothing to stop you from rushing out to buy that product to take care of your problem. Often people buy a product without really knowing much about it. They don't realize that some over-the-counter products should not be taken with certain prescription drugs, and that some products should be avoided if you suffer from a particular disease. Discount pharmacies do have a pharmacist on duty, but most of the time he or she is out of view.

An important thing to keep in mind is that even though the pharmacist does not wait on you personally, he or she is there to answer any questions you might have about your medicine. Nowadays pharmacists learn things in college that we old-timers did not, such as clinical pharmacy. This is a practice in which a pharmacist actually goes with a doctor on rounds and discusses with him or her the medication that would be most appropriate for the patient.

Even though people know the pharmacist is there, they

sometimes feel too embarrassed to ask questions. That could be a very big mistake. Today, there are more medications, whether over-the-counter or prescription, than there were back in the days of the Corner Drugstore. We now are able to cure with medicine many diseases that years ago were considered untreatable. However, a new problem has developed as a result, and that is drug interaction. Drug interaction is the effect of combining two or more medicines, whether they be prescription or nonprescription drugs. The interaction of certain drugs can be dangerous, sometimes even resulting in hospitalization.

Drug interactions have become so much of a problem that pharmacies are starting to maintain patient profiles (just like your doctor's) to keep track of the medicines you take. That is why it is important to try to deal with the same pharmacy each time. The pharmacist will be able to check your records for all the prescription medicines that you are or have been using. If there is a problem, he or she can call your doctor immediately. The pharmacist's records are especially important because this is an age of specialization and you may see different doctors for different reasons. For example, for a skin problem you may go to a dermatologist, for female problems to an obstetrician/gynecologist. Oftentimes they will prescribe a medicine for you; if they don't know that you are taking other medication, you could have a problem. If you deal with the same pharmacy each time, your pharmacist will be able to notice an incompatibility of drugs before you start taking a new medicine.

However it is also important to realize that over-the-counter medicines are drugs, too, and that problems may arise when they combine with prescription or other nonprescription drugs and even foods. I hope this book will serve as a valuable guide to over-the-counter drugs, explaining how and when they work, why some should not be used by certain people, and which should not be taken in combination with various substances.

Each chapter will cover a group of products found in the drugstore, such as laxatives, mouthwashes, shampoos, antacids, etc., grouped just as you would find them if you were looking for a product to buy. Every year there are more and more products on the market, each making its own individual claims. Of course, the manufacturers would like you to believe that their product is better than all the rest. However, no matter how many new products are produced and marketed, all usually have one thing in common: they usually have the same ingredients.

So in talking about the various products that are available, I have mentioned some common brand names, but mainly I talk about the ingredients in them and how they work. This will enable you, before you buy a new product, to check the ingredients to make sure they will take care of the symptoms you have, with the least number of side effects. The next step is to buy the cheapest product; as long as you have the right ingredients, it will work as well for you as a more expensive item.

So I hope that after reading this book you will know more about the products in the drugstore. And remember, if you have any questions about the product you are going to buy, ask your pharmacist. That is what he, or she, is there for—to help you make a safe and effective choice of products.

Now every home can have its own Corner Drugstore reference to help keep it on the road to good health, with useful information for every member of the family.

The Corner Drugstore

1

ACNE

ACNE is most common during the formative teenage years. Adolescence is a time for fun, friends, growing up, and—unfortunately—PIMPLES. While acne affects virtually everyone between the ages of thirteen and twenty-three, it may begin in females, due to hormonal changes, as early as ten or as late as the twenties or thirties. As evidenced by the many commercials on radio and television, competition for this multimillion-dollar market is keen among makers of acne medication. The large number of products—well over a hundred different ones are available —attests to the fact that there is no cure for acne. Yet, one should not be discouraged from treating the symptoms. Acne occurs most commonly on the face, back, and chest. Although it does not pose a severe physical threat, it should not be ignored, since it may cause a great deal of emotional stress and anguish. Contrary to popular belief, acne is not caused by such things as bad eating habits or poor hygiene, even though the eating of certain foods, uncleanliness, undue stress, and premenstrual tension may cause a flare-up of acne. The tendency to develop acne runs in families, especially those in which one or both parents have an OILY SKIN.

This problem sends people into the drugstore in droves to find products to clear up their acne. But there are so many products to pick from that you may not know where to start. The truth is that treatment will vary according to the severity and the type of acne.

Acne itself cannot be cured. In most cases, however, with currently available treatments, symptoms may be reduced and permanent scarring minimized. The best treatment is to remove excess oil from the skin, and this can be done very effectively by washing. The affected areas should be washed thoroughly three times a day with warm water, soap, and a soft washcloth. Scrubbing should be gentle to avoid damage and should be done for several minutes to work the lather thoroughly into the skin. The purpose of the washing is to produce a mild drying of the skin. However, if washing produces a feeling of tautness in the skin, its intensity and frequency should be reduced.

Ordinary facial soaps usually produce satisfactory results. Some soaps contain ingredients such as SULFUR and SALICYLIC ACID, but it is doubtful that these soaps are better, since if the affected area is rinsed properly, these added medications are washed away. If it is inconvenient to wash during the day, a cleansing pad that contains ALCOHOL or ACETONE may be used.

Since these treatments are aimed mainly at removing excess oil from the skin, other topically applied fats and oils—including most cosmetics—should be eliminated. Excessive amounts of hair dressings that contain oils should be avoided. Try to keep your hair short, because oily hair that comes in contact with your skin could cause further irritation of your acne condition. It is no matter which over-the-counter products you decide to try, for they all contain the same basic ingredients. So before you buy a product, read the label carefully. Look at the ingredients so you know how the product will work for you. Some products contain the following ingredients:

SULFUR

The main purpose of sulfur is to cut down the production of oil by the oil-producing glands. Sulfur is generally accepted as being an effective agent for improving the condition of acne. Products containing sulfur include CLEARASIL, CONTRABLEM, BENSULFOID, and ACNE-AID.

RESORCINOL AND SALICYLIC ACID

RESORCINOL and SALICYLIC ACID are used either separately or together in acne products. Both ingredients are used to remove dead, scaly tissue that builds up on the skin. A combination of resorcinol and salicylic acid in an alcoholic solution is very effective, because it dries quickly and does not leave a visible film on the skin. These ingredients are often added to products containing sulfur to increase its activity. A word of warning: Black people should try to avoid using products containing resorcinol, because it may produce a dark brown scale on the skin. These ingredients are found in the following over-the-counter products: ACNOMEL, CLEARASIL, CONTRABLEM, and DRY-AND-CLEAR acne medication and cream.

BENZOYL PEROXIDE

This is a very popular ingredient in acne medicines. It is found in products such as BENOXYL or OXY-5 and -10. BENZOYL PEROXIDE causes an increased sloughing rate, which in turn peels away skin that blocks the pores that produce oil. By opening the pores and letting the oil out, it prevents the formation of pimples. Benzoyl peroxide is used in concentrations of five and ten percent. The lower concentration is best to use if you are beginning treatment. It is usually applied at night after the affected area has been washed with soap and water. Fair-skinned people may find it to their advantage to leave it on for only two hours at a time until the skin becomes conditioned to the treatment.

BENZOYL PEROXIDE produces a feeling of warmth and stinging when applied to the skin and can even cause the skin to turn red. If the STINGING and BURNING sensation is too strong, remove the medicine immediately with soap and water and do not reapply it until the next day. Since this ingredient is highly IRRITATING, avoid contact with the eyes, lips, and neck. If you are using other methods of treatment, such as sun lamps, do not use them together since either may irritate the skin, and in combination could cause serious damage. Also avoid getting any of these products on your clothes, as they may bleach them. Then you'll have Mom to answer to, in addition to your acne.

The important thing to remember is that everyone goes through an acne period in their life. It is part of growing up. Unfortunately some people are affected more than others. There is no cure for acne. But adequate control can prevent permanent SCARRING, both physical and emotional. Dietary restriction is probably the most over-emphasized and least effective of the more widely used treatments for acne. Chocolate, nuts, carbonated soft drinks, and fried foods may contribute to acne. It is suggested that you avoid these foods for three weeks, then eat and drink them. If there is no change in your acne, then don't concern yourself with the diet. If you do notice a particular food or drink that causes your acne to flare up, then simply avoid it.

2

ALCOHOL

Nowadays many of the larger drugstores have a liquor section. And I must admit it does a goodly amount of business. Right away you are probably thinking, "Now what bad things is he going to say about alcohol?" I am not going to talk about your drinking habits—after all, you know them best. What I do want to tell you is that ALCOHOL is a drug, and an extremely active one. It is a central nervous system depressant and when combined with certain chemicals can cause undesirable problems. Although consumers may be wary of drinking when taking a prescription drug, they may not be so cautious when it comes to taking milder, nonprescription products. Many popular cough and cold remedies contain ANTIHISTAMINES; some also contain alcohol. Antihistamines, which also are used to treat allergies and to prevent motion sickness, have a tendency to cause drowsiness and to lessen coordination. Anyone who plans to treat a cold with a hot toddy and an over-the-counter antihistamine product will increase their drowsiness and make driving or operating machinery very hazardous.

Another popular over-the-counter drug is ASPIRIN, which has been a stand-by for treating HANGOVER. However, aspirin is very irritating to the stomach. When we drink alcohol, we wash away the stomach's protective coating, making it more susceptible to the irritating effects of aspirin. In general, then, it is not a bad idea to ask your pharmacist whether you can drink alcohol with any of the over-the-counter medicines you are taking, especially if you are not sure of the ingredients in the products you are taking or are about to buy.

Many people are in alcohol rehabilitation programs and may take medicines to lessen their craving for alcohol. If alcohol does come into contact with this medicine, it causes a reaction that ranges from NAUSEA and VOMITING to SHORT-NESS OF BREATH. While people who are intent on breaking their alcohol habit will avoid drinking, they may not realize that many products, especially cough syrups, contain an alcoholic base. For example, these popular cough remedies contain the following amounts of alcohol:

- BRONCHO-TUSSIN   40%   (80 proof)
- HALLS   22%   (44 proof)
- NYQUIL   25%   (50 proof)
- QUIET-NITE   25%   (50 proof)

The important thing to remember when buying any product is this: Check the ingredients thoroughly and make sure it does not contain alcohol. If you're not sure, ask the pharmacist. If you are sincere about kicking the drinking habit, you will take these steps.

One question people ask us pharmacists is: What is a safe amount of alcohol to drink provided you are not taking any medication? In order to measure the amount of alcohol in the blood, a blood test can be taken called a BAC (Blood Alcohol Concentration). But how do we know, when we are having a few drinks, how much alcohol is actually in the bloodstream? There is a rule of thumb that most people can go by, based on how many drinks you consume in a given amount of time and how much you weigh.

The following is a chart showing how many drinks are

required for persons of various weights to become intoxicated. Follow the chart closely to see what your limits are.

BODY WEIGHT (in pounds)		Number of Drinks (1½ ounces whiskey or 12 ounces beer) in a Two-Hour Period		
		Area 1	Area 2	Area 3
	100	1-2	3-4	5-12
	120	1-2	3-4	5-12
	140	1-2	3-4	5-12
	160	1-2	3-5	6-12
	180	1-2	3-5	6-12
	200	1-3	4-5	6-12
	220	1-3	4-6	7-12
	240	1-3	4-6	7-12

Area 1—Blood Alcohol Content up to 0.05% (Caution Required)
Area 2—Blood Alcohol Content above 0.05% (Driving Impaired)
Area 3—Blood Alcohol Content 0.10% or more (Driver Intoxicated)

However, remember one thing: The risk of intoxication increases if you are taking certain kinds of medication, whether over-the-counter products that contain antihistamines, such as cold remedies and sleeping aids, or prescription tranquilizers and sleeping pills.

3

ALLERGIES

There are approximately 35 million Americans in the United States who suffer from ALLERGIES. As a matter of fact, some people suffer from allergic reactions and don't even know it. They have symptoms of allergies but either ignore them or blame them on other things, such as a cold or sinus problems. UPSET STOMACHS, frequent HEADACHES, and DRY, ITCHY SKIN may all be symptoms of allergic reactions.

Allergies are reactions in our bodies to fight off foreign invaders. When this happens our body releases a substance called *histamine*. It is this histamine that causes symptoms like ITCHY, WATERY EYES, CONGESTION, and SWELLING of the mucous membranes, even RASHES. It is to counter this reaction that we take ANTIHISTAMINE.

Some products on the market, such as CHLOR-TRIME-TON or DIMETANE, are straight antihistamines. These products work very well to relieve allergic symptoms. These products have a side effect of DROWSINESS and SLEEPINESS, so use them with caution if you are driving a car or if you are engaged in some other activity that requires mental alertness. You should also try to avoid mixing these products with prescription medicines like tranquilizers or sleeping pills. Avoid alcohol since it is a depressant and when combined with antihistamines will cause excessive drowsiness. Antihistamines may have the opposite effect in children and elderly people and cause them to become nervous and over-excited.

Some over-the-counter products, including ALLEREST, CHLOR-TRIMETON decongestant, and CORICIDIN "D," contain both an antihistamine and a decongestant. While the antihistamine is working to relieve the itching and runny nose, it may cause the nose to become dry and clogged up, and the decongestant works very well to keep the nasal passages clear.

Some products, aside from having an antihistamine and decongestant in them, also have something in them for pain, such as ASPIRIN. Among these are BAYER DECONGESTANT, DRISTAN, or SINE-OFF. Other products, such as SINUTAB, CO TYLENOL, and SINAREST, contain an antihistamine, decongestant, and non-aspirin pain reliever. Since these products all contain a pain reliever, obviously the only people who should take them are those with a headache or pain due to sinus pressure. If an unfamiliar ingredient is listed on the package, ask the pharmacist about it. If you don't need it, don't buy the product. Just remember that the most commonly used pain relievers are ASPIRIN, ACETAMINOPHEN, and SALICYLAMIDE. Antihistamines usually found in these products are CHLORPHENIRAMINE, PHENIRAMINE, DOXYLAMINE, BROMPHENIRAMINE, PYRILAMINE, and PHENYLTOLOXAMINE. Common decongestants are PHENYLPROPANOLAMINE, PHENYLEPHRINE, EPHEDRINE, and PSEUDOEPHEDRINE.

Now it's just a matter of selecting the right product to treat the symptoms you have, and after that of finding the least expensive one.

COLDS AND HAY FEVER

People often come down with colds in the late summer that seem to hang around forever. These may be caused by allergies. Allergies also develop in the spring when the mild temperatures cause the trees and grasses to start pollinating. Unfortunately we notice it when we come out of a long winter hibernation and start working around the yard or cutting the grass. We usually end up sneezing our heads off. If pollen bothers you, you will notice that you feel better on rainy days, because the rain washes the pollen out of the air. Generally people suffering from these allergies feel worse during the morning hours.

If you enjoy working around the yard but don't enjoy the aggravation of SNEEZING and having ITCHY, WATERY EYES, you might try one of two things. Water your plants or grass at night, when they aren't pollinating, or wear a pollen mask, which is available at drugstores, to avoid breathing in the pollen.

Two other things that may cause you misery are mold and mildew, which grow outdoors on dead leaves and wet grass. Indoors, a damp basement, an unvented clothes dryer, and household plants are good places for them to grow. Mold and mildew can cause NASAL CONGESTION and even trigger an ASTHMA ATTACK. Allergic reactions to mold and mildew are most common in the evening hours, especially on damp evenings. They are not so common during the day because the sun dries the ground and grasses, thereby stopping mold growth.

OTHER ALLERGIES

Physical contact with certain substances may cause an allergic reaction of the skin. These substances include just about everything and range from the chemicals found in jewelry and cosmetics to those found in detergents. A very common cause of allergic RASHES is contact with plants such as poison ivy, poison oak, and poison sumac. (Turn to Chapter 39 for further information about poison ivy.)

Dust, insects, foods, medications, cigarette smoke, animal

fur, and feathers can all cause allergies by triggering various types of reactions in our bodies. Allergic reactions can even be fatal. Some appear on the skin in the form of RASHES or HIVES; some affect the respiratory tract, resulting in ITCHY, WATERY EYES, SNEEZING, and NASAL CONGESTION. Many mild forms of allergy can be controlled by avoiding the irritating substance. The use of medicines containing antihistamines or decongestants can help give you relief from the symptoms. For more severe allergies, a series of desensitizing injections can reduce or even eliminate the allergic reaction.

MILK ALLERGY

A common complaint among kids is a stomachache in the morning before getting onto the school bus. Recently doctors found that the cause of such recurring stomachaches in children is their inability to digest the sugar in milk. This condition sometimes occurs in adults as well. As a matter of fact, people who have drunk milk all their lives without a problem may suddenly notice that they develop CRAMPS, GAS, and even DIARRHEA when they drink milk. However, because we rely on milk for its CALCIUM, we can't just cut it out of our diets. Fortunately, there is a product on the market that makes the milk easier to digest. It is called LACTAID, and it does what your own body should do, which is to "split" the LACTOSE into its normal digestible form, without interfering with the taste of the milk.

This product is available in liquid and powder form. Simply add it to a quart of fresh milk and leave it in the refrigerator for about 24 hours. After this period of time, about 70 percent of the sugars in the milk are broken down. LACTAID works quite well in fresh skim or whole milk, powdered milk, or canned milk. The milk may be homogenized or not. It is not recommended for use in chocolate milk, although chocolate may be added after treatment. Be sure if you use whole milk that it is fresh, as the enzyme in this product does not work in buttermilk or other cultured products.

Many children and elderly adults develop this allergy to milk. If you are not sure whether you have this problem, it is very easy to find out. If you notice cramping, gas, or diarrhea after you drink milk, discontinue the use of all dairy products for 24 to 48 hours. If the symptoms disappear, there is a good chance that you have an allergic reaction to milk.

If you suspect that this is so, ask your doctor before you buy LactAid. He or she knows your medical background best. And if your pharmacist doesn't stock the item because it is new, ask him or her to order it for you.

4

ANTACIDS

One area of the Corner Drugstore that we all have visited at one time or another is the area that contains the ANT-ACIDS. Every year Americans spend millions of dollars on antacid products to relieve ACID INDIGESTION and HEART BURN from periodic bouts of overeating or -drinking. It seems that you can hardly watch television or pick up a magazine without seeing an ad of some kind for an antacid product that claims to do wonders for your indigestion. With lifestyles the way they are nowadays, eating on the run is a part of everyday living, and indigestion is the unwelcome "fringe benefit."

But before you buy an over-the-counter antacid, there are some things you should consider: How long have you had acid indigestion? Where is the pain located and when does it occur? Is it immediately, or several hours, after a meal? Is the pain relieved by food? Is it aggravated by coffee, carbonated beverages, or smoking? Are you taking medication, or has your doctor put you on a salt-free diet, or is he treating you for HIGH BLOOD PRESSURE? Answering these questions will help you select the right antacid and avoid causing additional problems.

Antacids are basically grouped into three types. The *coat-*

ing antacid has ingredients to coat and soothe the irritated walls of the stomach and to absorb excess stomach acid. The *effervescent* antacid, such as ALKA-SELTZER, neutralizes stomach acid. (These two are *basic* in nature and combine with the acid to neutralize it, which in turn relieves the discomfort.) The third type of antacid is one that has the ingredients of the coating antacids but has an additional ingredient for GAS. Thus it is important to know what some of the ingredients found in the antacids are and what they are intended to do.

SODIUM BICARBONATE

This is found in some of the most popular antacids on the market such as ALKA-SELTZER, DEWITT'S ANTACID POWDER, BELL-ANS BISODOL, SODA MINT, BROMO SELTZER, and ENO POWDER. Sodium bicarbonate is a potent antacid effective mainly for the relief of symptoms of occasional overeating or indigestion. Products containing sodium bicarbonate are not intended to be used for long periods of time, because they can eventually overload our system with SODIUM. This is extremely important for people who suffer from high blood pressure, since sodium may be the culprit in raising it in the first place. It is for this reason that doctors prescribe salt-free diets for patients with HIGH BLOOD PRESSURE (salt is the chemical compound SODIUM CHLORIDE).

ALUMINUM

Aluminum is usually found in antacid products as either ALUMINUM HYDROXIDE, ALUMINUM CARBONATE, or ALUMINUM PHOSPHATE. Of the three, aluminum hydroxide has the greatest neutralizing capacity. Aluminum hydroxide is found in products like AMPHOJEL, which is an ALUMINUM HYDROXIDE GEL. ALUMINUM CARBONATE is found in BAS-

ALGEL, and ALUMINUM PHOSPHATE is found in PHOSPHAL-JEL. The main side effect of aluminum antacids is CONSTI-PATION. Sometimes in elderly persons, since their intestinal movements are slower anyway, intestinal obstructions may develop. This constipative effect may be avoided by combining aluminum with MAGNESIUM SALTS, or by administering laxatives and stool softeners.

MAGNESIUM

Salts of magnesium that are commonly used in antacids are MAGNESIUM OXIDE, MAGNESIUM CARBONATE, MAGNESIUM HYDROXIDE, and MAGNESIUM TRESILICATE; of these the first three are the most potent. Magnesium salts are found in PHILLIPS' MILK OF MAGNESIA. Usually one teaspoonful is suitable for an antacid, but one tablespoonful is a laxative dose. Not surprisingly the most common side effect of magnesium is diarrhea. Probably the best antacids on the market are combinations of ALUMINUM and MAGNESIUM, such as ALUDROX, GELUSIL, MAALOX, or CAMA-LOX. Both are very good neutralizers of stomach acid, and aluminum offsets the side effects of magnesium, while magnesium offsets the side effects of aluminum.

CALCIUM CARBONATE

CALCIUM CARBONATE is also found in some antacids. It works fast and for a long period of time. Calcium carbonate is found in TITRALAC, liquid and tablets. The primary side effect of calcium antacids is CONSTIPATION. Also, too much calcium usage may result in the formation of kidney stones. Calcium antacids therefore should not be used for chronic stomach problems like ulcers. If consumed for more than a week or so, calcium may also cause "acid rebound," or the production of excess stomach acid, which could further irritate an ULCER. No matter what brand of antacid you use, it is usually available in tablet and liquid form. Do both work equally well? The liquid, because it is a liquid, absorbs more stomach acid. But the tablets are more convenient to carry around. If you want them to work as fast as the liquid, be sure to chew them up well and follow with water. Oftentimes people suck on them. Of course, it is not wrong, but they don't work as quickly that way. The problem is not in your mouth, it's in your stomach; so get the medicine down as quickly as you can.

GAS-RELIEVING ANTACIDS

The next group of antacids contain an additional ingredient to relieve GAS. The most common is called SIMETHICONE and is found in products like MAALOX PLUS, MYLANTA, and DI-GEL.

Simethicone causes gas bubbles to be broken down into a form that can be eliminated more easily by belching or passing gas. Simethicone itself is not an antacid, but combined with an antacid preparation, it makes a good, complete product for stomach distress. If your problem is *strictly* gas, you can buy a product like MYLICON, which is straight simethicone without the antacid portion.

Remember that not all antacids are equal, so you must know what you want your antacid to do. Large chain stores may carry their own brands of antacid. Compare their ingredients with the ingredients in the product you normally buy and you will probably notice that the only difference is in the price. Unless you like paying for the commercials you watch, buy the store brand. The money you save will be your own.

EFFERVESCENT ANTACIDS

The effervescent antacids work very rapidly to give us relief, but should not be used for chronic stomach problems.

The effervescent antacid that we are all familiar with is ALKA-SELTZER, which is now available in two varieties. What is the difference? ALKA-SELTZER in the blue package contains five grains of aspirin, ALKA-SELTZER in the gold package contains none. So if you have a headache along with your upset stomach, the blue may be effective. But remember that aspirin itself sometimes upsets the stomach.

A big problem with over-the-counter antacids is their possible interaction with prescription drugs. Antacids containing aluminum, calcium, and magnesium should not be combined with a certain group of antibiotics called the TETRACYCLINES. These chemicals combine with the tetracycline and cause it not to be absorbed properly. If you must take the two together, ask your doctor if you should space the doses, taking, for example, the tetracycline one hour before the antacid. IRON products should not be given with antacids because they decrease the body's ability to absorb the iron properly. Also, certain heart medications such as DIGOXIN and DIGITOXIN may be absorbed into the antacid that has coated our stomach, preventing it from being released into our system.

Some people who suffer from PARKINSON'S DISEASE take a drug called LEVODOPA. Unlike the other drug interactions, antacids may cause increased absorption of levodopa when the two are taken together. In general, since antacids work by either coating the stomach or neutralizing the acid in the stomach, taking any other medication—especially simultaneously—could be dangerous. To be on the safe side, before your doctor writes your prescription, or at the time you are getting it filled, tell your doctor or pharmacist that you take an antacid regularly.

However, no matter what type of antacid you use, here are some things to keep in mind: When using antacids to relieve indigestion, do not take them for longer than two weeks. If you don't get relief in this period of time, check with your doctor. When taking antacids, you should be aware they may cause DIARRHEA or CONSTIPATION. Patients on salt-free diets should avoid certain antacids because of their high SODIUM content. All antacids are not the same, and the failure of an antacid to treat your condition could be due to poor selection, taking it at the wrong time, or not taking the proper dose.

ANTACIDS FOR DIABETICS

Most of the well-known and widely used antacids, both liquids and tablets, contain sugar. Since sugar is an "inactive" ingredient, it is not listed on the label. Sugar-free products are available, however: BASALJEL, CAMALOX GELUSIL, MAALOX THERAPEUTIC CONCENTRATE, MAALOX PLUS, PHOSPHALJEL, RIOPAN, RIOPAN PLUS, SILAINGEL, and TRISOGEL. Most of these contain saccharin, but a few, Maalox Therapeutic Concentrate, Phosphaljel liquid, and Trisogel tablets, are free of both sugar and saccharin. All forms of ALUDROX, AMPHOJEL, GAVISCON, and MYLANTA contain sugar.

5

ASTHMA TIPS

ASTHMA is a disease of the respiratory system—that system of passageways that carries air from the nose and mouth to the lungs. The chief feature of asthma is DIFFICULT BREATHING, often accompanied by a WHEEZING or WHISTLING SOUND during exhalation. Asthmatic attacks occur at varying intervals. Between attacks, asthmatics are usually completely free of respiratory symptoms.

During an asthmatic attack the lining of the airways becomes CONGESTED and SWOLLEN and secretes excess mucus, which adds to the obstruction of the air flow. Asthma is an over-reaction of the respiratory system to any one or a combination of things, mainly—

- allergy-producing substances (allergens)
- respiratory infections
- emotional stress

Allergic asthma is seen most often in children. When it occurs, usually in the spring and summer, the cause of the allergy, and thus of the asthmatic attacks, is usually pollen or mold. When allergic asthma does not follow a seasonal pattern, it is usually caused by dust, animal dander, food, or drugs.

Respiratory infections are responsible for the development of asthmatic attacks in about 40 percent of asthmatics, usually middle-aged or older people, although this is also true for some youngsters. This type of asthma may also be seasonal, but this time the season is winter, when the greatest number of respiratory infections occur.

Emotional stress, and no other detectable reason, appears to be the trigger for about one-third of all asthmatic attacks. In children the start of a new school term, the birth of a brother or sister, or a separation from the parents may be the emotional trigger. In adults, a wide variety of family- or job-related problems may provoke an attack.

Preventive measures are usually directed toward the specific cause of the asthmatic attacks, for example, eliminating the offending allergen from the environment of the asthmatic. If the cause of asthma is animal dander, get rid of feather- or hair-stuffed pillows, mattresses, quilts, etc. Occasionally, a family pet may be the cause. If this is so, it may be necessary to find a new home for the bird or animal.

If dust is the offender, there are many ways to make your home as dust-free as possible. The center of attention in such cases should be the asthmatic's bedroom. After all, a child spends nearly half his life in his bedroom, while an adult normally passes about one-third of his time there. Here's what to do:

- Use smooth, not fuzzy, washable blankets and bedspreads.
- Do not use upholstered furniture.
- Use light, washable cotton or synthetic-fiber curtains rather than drapes.
- Use washable cotton throw rugs rather than wall-to-wall carpeting.
- Eliminate stuffed toys.

- Clean the room daily by damp dusting and damp mopping.
- Keep the door closed.

Vacuuming blows a great deal of dust into the air, so don't vacuum in the presence of an asthmatic person. If you are asthmatic, try to get someone else to do this chore. Also remember that the chemical irritants in many cleaning products used at home are generally taboo for asthmatics.

If pollen is the offender, an air conditioner with a filter should be installed in the asthmatic's room and sometimes the entire home. Obviously, long walks in the country are out during high pollen periods. Sometimes it is impossible to get away from an air-borne allergen such as pollen. In these cases a doctor may try a technique called DESENSITIZATION.

If a specific food is the cause, obviously it should not be eaten. Likewise, certain drugs are known to trigger asthmatic attacks in susceptible individuals. Among the most common offenders are ASPIRIN and aspirin-containing compounds.

The following list of do's and don'ts should prove very helpful:

- Don't smoke and don't stay in a room with people who do, whether it is at home, at a business, or in a public place.
- Do stay away if your home is being painted. Paint fumes are notorious for provoking asthmatic attacks.
- Do avoid sudden changes of temperature. Don't wander in and out of air-conditioned stores on a hot summer's day.
- Don't go outside in extremely cold weather. If you must, a cold-weather mask may be helpful.
- Do avoid people with respiratory infections whenever possible.
- Do try to avoid emotionally upsetting situations.

- Do get enough fluid in your diet—six to eight glasses of liquids a day.
- Don't over-exert yourself. But don't stay away from all exercise either. Be your own best guide as to how much activity you can tolerate. Schedule frequent rest periods if you know you're going to have a busy day.
- Don't take any medicine without telling your doctor. This includes simple remedies you can buy without a prescription. Remember that even aspirin can cause asthma.
- Do take all medications prescribed by your doctor exactly as directed.
- Don't take sleeping pills or sedatives if you can't sleep because of a mild asthma attack. These medications have a tendency to slow down your breathing and make breathing more difficult. Instead try propping yourself up on extra pillows while waiting for your anti-asthma medication to work.
- Avoid inhalation of insecticides, deodorants and cleaning aids, etc.
- If a severe attack develops, get medical help immediately.

Some people who suffer from chronic lung problems like asthma use the portable aerosol products, such as PRIMATENE MIST or BRONKAID MIST. These products work fairly well. The active ingredient is EPINEPHRINE, which is responsible for dilating the bronchioles so that you can breathe easier.

There are some other over-the-counter medicines that can be used to treat people suffering from asthma. These products differ from the cold remedies in that they contain ingredients to open up the bronchioles. EPHEDRINE has been used for a number of years and is found in products like AMODRINE, TEDRAL, BRONKAID, BRONKOTABS, and PRIMATENE P.

EPHEDRINE is effective in clearing the bronchioles to allow you to breathe easier. However, tolerance to the drug develops with frequently repeated doses, causing your body to need more and more of the drug in order for it to work properly. Overuse of products with ephedrine in them can cause NERVOUSNESS, TREMORS, and INSOMNIA. They can also cause the heart to speed up and even elevate the blood pressure.

Products with ephedrine are slow in taking effect, but act for a long period of time. These products are mainly useful to people who have milder forms of asthma. Since they can affect sugar levels in the bloodstream, diabetics should monitor their urine sugar levels closely. Caution is advised for older male patients with PROSTRATE PROBLEMS, because urinary retention may occur.

These products contain an additional ingredient called THEOPHYLLINE, which is also found in BRONITIN, BRONK-AID, TEDRAL, and BRONKOTABS. Theophylline causes relaxation of the muscles of the bronchioles. Theophylline and ephedrine can cause excessive stimulation of the central nervous system, which is why some manufacturers have added a sedative, such as PHENOBARBITAL, to their products. Another main side effect of theophylline is that it causes irritation of the stomach. If these products do upset your stomach, try taking them with food or milk.

It is important to take your medicine routinely to prevent an asthma attack. If you notice that your attacks are occurring more frequently, check with your doctor: You may need a different type of medication or one that is only available by prescription.

EPINEPHRINE is another ingredient used to treat people suffering from asthma. However, it is only effective when taken by injection or by inhalation, because it is destroyed by the gastric juices of the stomach. All over-the-counter aerosol products used for asthma contain epinephrine or one of its salt forms, including ASTHMA NEFRIN, BREATHEASY, BRONKAID MIST, and PRIMATENE MIST. There are relatively few side effects with these products, because they are inhaled and very little is absorbed into your system. However, overuse can produce side effects such as NERVOUSNESS, TREMORS, RESTLESSNESS, and PALPITATIONS. Sometimes people using these products develop a DRY MOUTH and THROAT. These side effects can be alleviated by gargling after each use.

There are many problems with these products: When we have an asthma attack we are prone to panic, and so we may spray the mist into our mouths several times. However, these products sometimes cause further irritation to the bronchioles. Remember to spray only once—you will get relief just as fast, without complications.

EPINEPHRINE, the active ingredient in these products, is readily destroyed by light or heat, so if you do use these products, store them in a cool, dark place so that they are ready to work for you when seconds really count.

6

BOTTLED WATERS

More and more drug stores are carrying bottled waters, but all bottled waters are not equal. Some are carbonated and some are not, some are natural and others processed. Some taste refreshing and pure, others taste like medicine. One thing is sure: They are not cheap. As a rule, you will pay more for imported waters than for domestic brands. In either case, it is important to know what you want the bottled water to do for you and then to read the label carefully to make sure that it does it.

Many people prefer bottled waters to tap water because of the taste. Others are concerned about the chemicals put into our drinking water to purify it. Some people drink bottled waters for health reasons, because some brands are high in mineral content.

Below are the types of water that are bottled. All are pure, but not all come from natural springs. Many American brands are simply bottled tap or well water that has been chemically treated or purified. They use terms on their labels like "spring-fresh," "spring-pure," or "formulated"; these words mean that the water you are buying is not natural. Another description that appears on the label of bottled waters is "natural spring water," which means that it comes to the earth's surface by its own force without being pumped out. Such water is naturally rich in VITAMINS and MINERALS. There are two types of natural spring water and they are still, or noncarbonated, and carbonated with natural gases from the ground. The advantage of natural carbonation is that it stays in the liquid for a longer period of time than added carbonation does.

- **Processed or Treated Water**—These words stated on the label mean that your water comes from a stream, or a well, or even a tap. It is then put through a purification process, during which chemicals and minerals are added or removed to improve the taste.
- **Well Water**—This is water that must be pumped to reach the earth's surface. It is usually processed for bottling.
- **Fluoridated Water**—This term simply means that the water contains controlled amounts of FLUORIDE to help prevent TOOTH DECAY in children. This water is useful if you live in rural areas where fluoride is not added to the water. Cities usually have fluoride added to their water supplies.
- **Distilled Water**—This is water that has no minerals because it has gone through a process in which the water is changed to a vapor and then converted back to a liquid. It has no flavor. It is the type of water used in irons or humidifiers, because it doesn't create a build-up of chemicals that hampers their working.

So if you do use bottled waters, or if you are considering using them, these are the sorts of information to look for on the label. Make sure you are getting the product that you want and that will do the best job for you, especially at those prices!

7

COLD REMEDIES

In life two things are inevitable: taxes and colds. Although symptoms for the common cold and allergies are similar, they are caused by different things. Nearly every company advertises the "right product to treat your problem"—one reason why cold remedies compose one of the largest areas of the Corner Drugstore. Some of the products that are available contain a number of different ingredients, many of which we don't really need, and some of which can cause further complications. Some cold remedies are claimed to have ingredients to treat twenty cold symptoms. In fact, one of the main ingredients in these products is plain ASPIRIN, which will relieve ten cold symptoms all by itself.

Before buying any cold remedy you should ask yourself what symptoms you have: RUNNY NOSE, SORE THROAT, COUGH, FEVER, EARACHE? Answering these questions will help you select the right product.

Also consider how long you have had your symptoms. Do you have a history of allergies or of respiratory diseases such as ASTHMA or BRONCHITIS? If you have DIABETES, GLAUCOMA, HEART DISEASE, THYROID problems, or HIGH BLOOD PRESSURE and are taking prescription drugs, then you should avoid certain over-the-counter medications. And finally, if your job requires mental alertness, certain over-the-counter medicines should be avoided because they cause DROWSINESS and may result in an accident or other dangerous situation.

The common cold is a mixture of symptoms affecting the upper respiratory tract. Usually the symptoms are caused by one of many viruses. The intensity of the symptoms may vary from hour to hour. Like any virus, a cold runs its course and leaves the body as quickly as it came. The only reasonable way to treat a cold is to alleviate the particular symptoms you have.

The common cold has been rated as the single most expensive illness in the United States. In fact, more time is lost from work and school because of the common cold than any other illness. Age is related to the incidence of the common cold. Children from one to five years old are most susceptible. Body chills or wet feet in themselves do not cause the common cold, but a sudden change in body temperature allows the virus to invade the body more easily. It is then that we develop cold symptoms and join the American public in spending approximately $500–700 million a year on over-the-counter cough, cold, and allergy products.

The following is an outline of the ingredients found in over-the-counter cold remedies. Simply compare the ingredients on the package with your symptoms and you will know whether that product will give you relief or merely waste your money.

ANTIHISTAMINES

Histamine is found in every body tissue. It is released from the tissues and into our system in both the common cold and allergies, causing ITCHY, WATERY EYES, SNEEZING, a RUNNY NOSE, even HIVES. **ANTIHISTAMINES** block the formation of histamine, and therefore prevent or relieve these allergy or cold symptoms. Some of the antihistamines most commonly found in over-the-counter products are CHLOR-

PHENIRAMINE, BROMPHENIRAMINE, DOXYLAMINE, METHAPYRILENE, PHENINDAMINE TARTRATE, PHENIRAMINE, and PYRILAMINE.

All these are antihistamines and relieve cold symptoms. But they are best suited for allergies. People who use antihistamines regularly sometimes find that they don't work as well as at first. This is because the presence of some antihistamines in the system causes the liver to produce enzymes at a faster rate to break down the antihistamines: That is, the body develops a tolerance for them.

Antihistamines may cause problems with a cold because they produce a drying effect. If you have CONGESTION the antihistamine thickens and hardens the mucus, making it difficult to clear the upper respiratory passages. That is why many cold remedies contain both an antihistamine and decongestant; as the antihistamine dries you up, the decongestant keeps the sinuses open.

At recommended doses, most over-the-counter antihistamines are safe for use by children. However, an accidental overdose in children may lead to side effects of excitement and muscle-twitching.

All antihistamines cause DROWSINESS, but the degree of drowsiness varies with the antihistamine. People should be careful not to combine them with tranquilizers or alcohol, which also cause drowsiness. The combination could be dangerous, especially if you have to operate any type of machinery or if your job requires you to be alert.

Antihistamines may also react with birth control pills, because antihistamines cause the body to produce enzymes that break down certain chemicals in the body. One of the ingredients in birth control pills is a female hormone called ESTRADIOL, which is affected by the enzymes produced by antihistamines, causing the pill to be less effective. You may develop unusual bleeding or spotting; it may even cause frequent or irregular periods.

The point is, whether you are just starting to take birth control pills, or have been taking them for a while, let your doctor know if you notice any changes in your monthly cycle. He can prescribe a stronger birth control pill to counter the effects of the antihistamine, especially if you have to take these products frequently.

Other common side effects of antihistamines are dry mouth, blurred vision, and urinary problems. People with GLAUCOMA should also try to avoid antihistamines, or use them under a doctor's supervision.

If you suffer from allergic reactions to plants, such as poison ivy, or insect bites, oral antihistamines will help relieve the itching and discomfort caused by these things. Some topical treatments for itching contain antihistamines, but since absorption is poor through the skin, you will find that oral products like CHLOR-TRIMETON and DIMETANE work much better.

DECONGESTANTS

Decongestants are probably the most useful ingredients in over-the-counter cold remedies. These products constrict the blood vessels, which in turn opens up the sinuses, so that we can breathe more easily.

Common decongestants are PHENYLPROPANOLAMINE, PHENYLEPHRINE, and PSEUDOEPHEDRINE.

Many products contain decongestants along with antihistamines or pain relievers; however, some products, like SUDAFED, are just straight decongestants.

There are several side effects of decongestants: one is ELEVATION OF BLOOD PRESSURE as a result of the constriction of the blood vessels. If you suffer from high blood pressure and wish to take a decongestant, you should be aware of their effect. If you are taking prescription medication to control your high blood pressure, taking decongestants may counteract your medicine.

Decongestants stimulate the central nervous system, which may result in SLEEPLESSNESS. This side effect often helps offset the drowsiness caused by antihistamines.

Because they stimulate the heart, decongestants may

cause CARDIAC ARRYTHMIAS. So be careful when using products containing the ingredients mentioned earlier. Even though you can buy them without a prescription, stop taking them and call your doctor if you notice anything unusual.

TOPICAL DECONGESTANTS

Topical decongestants are more commonly known as nose sprays. They contain the same ingredients as the oral products but are sprayed directly into the nose. They work well; after spraying the nose opens up and we breathe freely. However, there is a danger that because they work so well, we will begin using them all the time.

Nose sprays have a distressing side effect called NASAL REBOUND. That means that shortly after the nose is sprayed it clogs up again, not because of the cold, but because of the spray itself. Using the nose spray repeatedly to clear the nasal passages is likely to result in a vicious cycle of addiction. Even after your cold is gone, you will not be able to breathe freely without the aid of decongestant sprays or liquids. This turn of events may very well make the manufacturers of these products happy, but it is both expensive and unhealthy for you. Excessive use of nose sprays also causes the nose to bleed more easily. Their one advantage is that, since they are not taken orally, they do not cause an increase in blood pressure.

If you have a bad cold and are taking a cold tablet but need additional relief, it is not wrong to use a nose spray. However, do not use it more than two or three times a day. I would recommend the long-acting sprays because they are intended to be used only twice a day. And when your cold is gone, take that nose spray and pitch it.

If you have become hooked on nose sprays, some doctors recommend the use of a salt solution to help heal the irritated sinuses. The solution consists of one-half teaspoonful baking soda and one teaspoonful salt dissolved in a quart of cool tap water. Fill an empty spray bottle half full of the freshly made solution and spray into the nose several times a day to flush out the sinuses. The first few days will be a little uncomfortable, but as the sinuses heal the swelling that causes congestion goes down and you can get rid of your nose spray for good.

COUGH SYRUPS

What's a cold without a cough? Actually a cough is a natural reflex of your body to help clear mucus out of the bronchioles. But when that cough becomes an aggravating tickle in the back of the throat, you want to get rid of it. This can be done in one of two ways. Usually the tickle is due to the throat being dried out from breathing through the mouth. A cough drop or even a piece of hard candy will lubricate it and stop the tickle. If you have a lot of head congestion, you may want to use a cough drop containing MENTHOL and CAMPHOR. While the cough drop moistens your throat, the menthol and camphor vapor help unclog the sinuses.

Cough syrups are more confusing. Many of them contain a mixture of antihistamines and decongestants. If you are already taking a cold tablet, you could be getting a "double whammy" of these drugs, bringing out their more serious side effects. Some cough syrups, such as NYQUIL, have alcoholic bases; as a matter of fact, NYQUIL has 25 percent alcohol, which makes it 50 proof. No wonder you sleep so well. However, there is reason to be concerned about the effect that an alcohol-based cough syrup has on former alcoholics.

Most cough products are either syrups or elixirs. Syrups have sugar bases, elixirs have alcohol bases. Either could have extremely dangerous consequences for a diabetic. Your pharmacist may be able to recommend a sugarless, nonalcoholic product.

Some cough syrups have an ingredient called DEXTRO-METHORPHAN, which is a cough suppressant and is somewhat effective in stopping a hacking, aggravating COUGH. But dextromethorphan can cause DROWSINESS and an UPSET

STOMACH. The other ingredients sometimes found in cough syrups, such as **ROBITUSSIN**, is GUIAFENESIN. This ingredient does not actually stop the cough reflex. It is most useful when you have congestion in the chest from thick mucus, because it breaks up the mucus and allows you to bring it up when you cough. However, if you have both a hacking cough and congestion, then the answer is obvious: Pick a cough syrup with a cough suppressant as well as an ingredient to loosen phlegm, like **ROBITUSSIN-DM, CHERACOL D,** or **PERTUSSIN Cough Syrup for Children.** The important thing to keep in mind, no matter what cough syrup you use, is this: If your cough persists for more than two or three days, don't fool around—check with your doctor. Respiratory infections are not things to be taken lightly.

Don't spend money foolishly on products that have many ingredients. Chances are you don't really need them. Some of the cold remedies and hay fever products are available in long-acting forms. You have no doubt seen the ads for the time-release pills that promise continuous relief for eight to twelve hours. If you expect them to work for everybody for that period of time, you have been fooled. No two individuals are alike, and many factors affect a person's ability to absorb medicines, including when you had your last meal. What lasts for one person for eight hours may only work for another for four hours. And if you begin taking more than you are supposed to, you could be causing additional problems for yourself.

If your cold continues to get worse even while you are taking your favorite cold remedy, or if you begin to run a temperature, be sure to call your doctor to get his advice. The duration of your cold depends on how soon you start treating it, and on using the right product.

COOL-AIR HUMIDIFIERS

Another way to cope with a cold is to use a cool-air humidifier. These machines spray a cool mist into the air, which lubricates the nose and throat and keeps the mucus moving so that it does not collect in one spot and cause congestion. Cool-air humidifiers are also useful even if you don't have a cold. Often times, especially during the cooler months when the heat is on, you may wake up in the morning with your nose and throat all dried out. This creates an environment receptive to viruses, which in turn causes colds.

When people go to a drugstore to buy a humidifier, they often are confused by all the different types. Remember that all cool-air humidifiers work the same way; the only difference is in the amount of water they hold, which in turn determines how long the unit will work without being refilled. If you use a cool-air humidifier, try to change the water each time you use it to avoid having mold develop. You certainly don't want *that* blowing all over your room! Also be sure to clean your humidifier periodically because the chemicals that are in the water can build up in your humidifier and hamper its performance.

STEAM VAPORIZERS

In the early days around the turn of the century, it wasn't uncommon in any home where a person was suffering from a respiratory disease, such as a cold or flu, to heat a pot or kettle of water with eucalyptus leaves in it. A towel was then placed over the pot and the vapors breathed in. The eucalyptus vapors helped open the sinuses.

Later on companies came out with a more sophisticated form of this old folk remedy, which was called a "vaporizer" and was electric. No longer was the water heated on a stove. The leaves were replaced by patented products, such as KAS and VICKS VAPO STEAM, that you could buy in a drugstore. But there was a potential hazard of a child or adult pulling over the vaporizer and causing a severe burn. Hot-air vaporizers are still being sold in drugstores, but they are a lot safer nowadays because they are available in units that cannot spill, even if they are accidentally knocked over.

Steam vaporizers are mainly used by people in order to

keep their noses open by breathing in inhalants. However, many doctors prefer the cool-air vaporizers. The moist cool air keeps the nose and throat passages coated so that mucus does not accumulate in one area, causing irritation.

FEVER

FEVER is a rise of body temperature above normal. If you look carefully, most thermometers have an arrow pointing to the mark for 98.6°, for this is the normal oral temperature, measured on the Fahrenheit scale.

Since everyone is different, normal temperatures will vary; some children will have a slightly higher normal temperature, and some slightly lower. Normal oral temperatures range from 97.7° to 99.5°F. It is also important to know that the body temperature of a healthy child is continually changing, going up a little or down a little, depending on the time of day and the activity of the child.

However, when your child's temperature reaches 101°F. or more, it is probably due to illness and you should call your doctor. This does not mean that you should ignore temperatures lower than 101°F. A persistent LOW-GRADE FEVER, where your child's temperature is continually a degree or two above normal, may also indicate the presence of illness and the need for the advice of a doctor. Here are some signs that will tell you when to take your child's temperature:

- Skin: hot, dry, excess sweating, rash
- Complexion: very pale or unusually flushed
- Cold Symptoms: runny nose, sneezing or coughing, hoarseness

It is also a good idea to check it if your child tells you he or she does not feel well.

Taking your child's temperature is usually a lot easier said than done. There are two basic types of thermometers, the oral and the rectal. The only difference is in the shape of the bulb on the end of each thermometer. The one on the rectal thermometer is round or oval. The bulb on the oral thermometer is slim and long. The markings on the two thermometers are the same.

Rectal thermometers are most often recommended for infants. Apply a little VASELINE to the bulb end, then insert it into the rectum about one-third of its length. It should move easily; never force a thermometer. Hold the thermometer in the rectum for about two or three minutes, then gently pull it out. Wipe off the thermometer with a tissue. In good light, slowly rotate the thermometer until you see the mercury. The normal temperature rectally is 99.6°F. After you have read the thermometer, wash it with cold or lukewarm, soapy water, wipe it with alcohol, and put it away in its container. Never use hot water.

When the child is one year or older, its better to take the temperature in the armpit, unless your doctor tells you otherwise. Place the bulb of the thermometer securely in the child's armpit and hold his arm across his chest. Allow the thermometer to remain there for three to four minutes. The normal temperature under the arm is 97.6°F. If you call your doctor when a child is sick, always tell him or her not only what the child's temperature is, but also the way you took it: orally, rectally, or under the arm.

Nowadays there are easier ways to take your child's temperature. Instead of a thermometer, there are small patches that you can stick to your child's forehead. They contain heat-sensitive colored crystals and, as the temperature changes, a different color shows up in the form of a number. Two products that are available in the drugstore and that work in this way are called STICK TEMP and EZ TEMP. The advantage of using these products, besides avoiding the wrestling act with the kids, is that once you stick it to the child's head, you can leave it there as long as she or he is ill. It will give a constant read-out of the body temperature.

So if you have trouble taking your child's temperature, try using one of these products. I think you'll find them very useful. They are quite accurate and even some hospitals are starting to use these sorts of fever thermometers.

Fever in itself is usually not dangerous, as long as it is not extremely high and lost body water is adequately replaced. In many instances, the best thing you can do for your child with a fever is to keep him cool. Here's how you can do this:

- Keep your child undressed in the house; the fewer the clothes, the faster the fever will go down.
- Do not cover your child with blankets or quilts in bed.
- Give lots of cool, clear liquids to your child. Do not give milk! Milk often upsets the stomach of a child with a fever.
- Give popsicles, ice water, sherbert, or carbonated beverages.
- Give cool sponge baths. (If temperature is over 102°F. set your child in a tub of tepid water.) Do not use alcohol. Sponge or pour water over the back and front for at least a half hour. Do not use cold water.
- Do not give your child an enema for fever. Enemas should be given on doctor's orders only.

FEVER BLISTERS

Colds come and go, but they sometimes leave behind a FEVER BLISTER. When we have a cold or fever, the lips become dry, which promotes the growth of the viruses that cause fever blisters. As a matter of fact, exposure to the sun sometimes causes fever blisters. Fever blisters are contagious for the first two to three days. Touching them and then touching another part of your body may cause them to spread.

There are some products available to treat fever blisters. First we have the drying agents such as SPIRITS OF CAM-

PHOR or CAMPHO-PHENIQUE. They help to dry up the fever blister. The problem with these products is that they cause the fever blister to form a hard scab; when you open your mouth, the fever blister is liable to crack open, causing bleeding and pain.

Some products coat the fever blister and keep it soft, such as the lip balms like CHAPSTICK, VASELINE INTENSIVE CARE lip balm, or BLISTIK. Some, like BLISTEX or BLISTR KLEAR, are in cream form.

There is even an oral product available called LYSINE TABLETS, which are available in 500 mg. tablets without a prescription. They are nothing more than an amino acid which is already present in our bodies in the form of protein. The usual dosage is three tablets a day for three to four days. Some people say it cuts down on the length of time they have a fever blister.

If you are frequently bothered by fever blisters, you might want to talk to your doctor about getting a smallpox vaccination. The virus that causes fever blisters is related to the virus that causes smallpox but is much weaker. Therefore if you have a smallpox vaccination, it may help stop the virus causing fever blisters. Talk to your doctor; he knows what is best for you.

8

CONTACT LENSES

Because of advances being made in the medical field today, more and more people are able to wear contact lenses. As improved contact lenses become available, they increasingly are being fitted as an alternative to eyeglasses for primary vision correction. Competition among lens manufacturers and practitioners has led to decreased lens cost, making contact lenses affordable to a larger segment of the population. Also, new lens designs allow people with specific vision problems requiring a certain type of lens to have access to contact lenses.

With so many people wearing contact lenses, let's talk about some things to keep in mind. Before handling the contact lenses or their case, be sure that your hands are clean. There are three general rules or goals that are important for the person who wears any type of contact lens.

- Keep the lenses clean. This should be done on a daily basis to remove mucus from the lens surface.
- Contact lenses should be kept in an antiseptic soaking solution when they are not in the eye.
- A wetting agent should be used to put the contact lens in the eye.

It is also important to clean the contact lens storage case on a regular basis—that is, every day or two. For hard contact lenses, use a mild soap or baking soda to clean the case, then let it air-dry. The soft lens storage case can be rinsed in hot tap water and then allowed to air-dry. Women may wear make-up with contacts, but should be careful if they wear soft lenses because these are easily penetrated by foreign substances. Mascara, make-up, and hair dyes can soak into the lens and ruin it. Foreign material on or under the lens will produce extreme discomfort. Care should be exercised by both the hard- and soft-lens wearer when using hair and deodorant sprays; these products should be used before the lenses are put in the eyes. Also, never administer eye drops to the eyes while the contacts are in place.

In the drugstore you will see many products to use with your contact lenses. The cleaning and wetting solutions are different for hard and soft lenses. It is very important not to use a hard contact lens solution with the soft lenses, because hard lens solutions contain a preservative called BENZAL-KONIUM CHLORIDE. This ingredient binds into the soft plastic and causes a burning sensation when the soft lens is put in the eye. If this happens to you, don't panic; it is uncomfortable, but it won't cause permanent eye damage.

HARD CONTACT LENSES

Hard contact lenses usually last about five years if you don't lose them, and provided you take special care of them. It is important to use the right solution on a hard contact lens, so be sure to read the information on the package thoroughly before you buy it. First of all there are the cleaning solutions such as BARNES-HINDS, LENSINE, and LC-65. A cleansing solution should be used on a daily basis. It removes mucus and debris that could cloud or fog up your lens. The other type of solution is a soaking solution and is available in such products as SOQUETTE, CONTIQUE, and SOAKCARE. When you are not wearing your contact lenses, be sure to use one of these solutions in the storage case; they contain an ingredient to kill bacteria that could cause eye infections. The third type of solution is the wetting solution, such as **BARNES-HIND'S WETTING SOLUTION, VISA-LENS,** and **LIQUIFILM.** These products are used directly on the lenses just before putting them in the eyes. Their main purpose is to make the lens more compatible with the eye and to keep the lens from stinging your eye when it is applied. If it stings anyway, wash the lens with water before you put it in. The wetting solutions contain a lubricant and these lubricants can burn the eye.

SOFT CONTACT LENSES

Soft contact lenses are a lot easier to get used to than hard ones—they are quite comfortable. With proper care, which usually takes two to three minutes a day, these contacts will last about two years.

Soft contacts are stored in a solution that is similar to our own natural tears. This salt solution was once prepared by using distilled water and special salt tablets. However, the F.D.A. has taken the tablets off the market, because they were often prepared under conditions that were not sterile and eye infections resulted. Now we have prepared solutions to store and disinfect the soft contact lenses. Products like **BOIL AND SOAK, LENSRINS,** and **SOFT THERM** are only intended to be used with the heat disinfectant. But there is a second method of disinfecting soft lenses, called the chemical or cold treatment. Check with your doctor before using this method, because the chemicals in the treatment cause reactions in certain people. Do not switch back and forth between cold and hot methods of disinfecting, because it could ruin the lens. Remember that soft lenses are more easily penetrated by mascara, eye make-up, and hair dyes.

Never place contacts in the mouth to wet them, and never wipe them with a cloth or tissue that could scratch the lens. When you go to your doctor be sure to tell him that you wear contact lenses before he writes out a prescription for you, because some drugs can dry out the eye. It also wouldn't be a bad idea to wear some sort of medical alert necklace or bracelet if you wear contact lenses.

Contact lenses are great—convenient, attractive, and effective. But remember when you get a pair to be sure to get all the information available regarding your lenses. Read the literature thoroughly. Knowing a lot about your lenses can prevent problems in the future. And if you are confused about which lens-care product to buy, ask your pharmacist to help you.

9

CONTRACEPTIVE PRODUCTS

Recent trends toward smaller families suggest that more and more people are using some sort of birth control method. As a matter of fact, many pharmacies are developing family planning centers in which personnel are available to answer questions and to show the different types of products that are on the market. Contraceptive products are available without prescription for both men and women.

CONDOMS

A condom is a contraceptive device used by males and is a very popular method of birth control. Condoms used to be kept behind the prescription counter, so that you had to ask the pharmacist for them. Men and women asked for them by a variety of names, such as bags, balloons, rubbers, safes, skins, and prophylactics. (I remember that once a fellow came into the drug store and asked for head gaskets for a hot rod. I didn't know what he was talking about. You guessed it—he wanted condoms.)

Nowadays, most drugstores have a display of condoms right out in the open. This has caused raised eyebrows among some people. The thing to keep in mind is that it was embarrassing for people to ask for condoms. Now they can be purchased without the anxiety of having to ask someone. Interestingly, women buy them more often than men. As a matter of fact, it is a good idea for women to carry them in their purses, because they cannot always depend on their male partner to supply adequate protection. Condoms are simple to use, harmless, inexpensive, and very effective. They offer two kinds of protection: against pregnancy and against venereal disease. As a matter of fact, they are the only contraceptive method that prevents V. D.

Condoms are usually made of rubber (latex), but some are made from animal intestine and are called "skins." Although they provide a high degree of protection against conception, accidents such as tearing or rupture of the condom do happen. Two techniques help prevent the condom from bursting: Let it extend about an inch beyond the end of the erect penis to hold the semen. If lubrication is necessary, use one of the water-soluble lubricants, such as K-Y JELLY. Never use VASELINE or any other petroleum product; they may react with the rubber and deteriorate it. Even though condoms are very effective, there are a number of pregnancies reported each year using these products. Be sure you know enough about the product before you buy it and if you have any questions, ask!

VAGINAL CONTRACEPTIVES

These contraceptives are applied vaginally. They are available in creams and gels, along with an applicator. You fill the applicator and insert it into the vagina. Also available are foams that are in aerosol containers and are accompanied by an applicator. The newest form is a suppository.

The choice depends on your personal preference: The creams provide greater lubrication during intercourse. The jelly is easier to remove because it is completely water-soluble and dissolves. Foams do not help lubricate but are undetectable during use. All of these products contain a spermicide to kill sperm.

Foams and creams designed to be used without a diaphragm are CONCEPTROL, DALKON, DELFEN, EMKO, LANTEEN, and RAMSES 10-HOUR. Vaginal contraceptives that are used with a diaphragm are KOROMEX II, ORTHO-CREME, and ORTHO-GYNOL. ENCARE and SEMICID are suppositories and, like the foams and jellies, contain a spermicide.

ENCARE OVAL effervesces when it is inserted to cover the area to be protected. To determine its freshness you can moisten it with a drop of water. If the tablet begins to bubble, insert it immediately. The main advantage of suppositories is that they are easier to use. With other vaginal contraceptives, you must deal with a tube and applicator, and sometimes a diaphragm; with the suppository, that's all there is.

Store all of these products in a cool, dry place and try to use them within a six-month period.

About ten to twenty pregnancies are reported for every 100 women using these products. This is simply because of misuse of these products. Whether you are using cream, foam, jelly, or suppository, it must be applied less than one hour before sexual intercourse and should remain in the vaginal tract for eight hours afterwards. Before each subsequent intercourse, an additional applicatorful or suppository should be inserted.

As with any applied chemical, irritation of the vagina and penis may occur. In that case, discontinue using the product and try another method.

DOUCHING

Flushing out the vagina immediately after intercourse to remove semen is an age-old method of attempting to avoid pregnancy. Unfortunately, this after-the-fact method is totally unreliable. The idea behind the practice is to remove the semen before it enters the uterus. However, sperm can reach the mouth of the uterus within 90 seconds after ejaculation. There are a number of douche products available: LYSETTE, MASSENGILL DISPOSABLE DOUCHE, MASSENGILL DOUCHE POWDER, MASSENGILL LIQUID, MASSENGILL VINEGAR AND WATER DISPOSABLE DOUCHE, NYLMERATE II, and TRICHOTINE liquid and powder. You can rely on them for hygienic purposes, not for contraception.

RHYTHM

The Rhythm Method is abstinence from sexual relations during the fertile period of the female cycle. It is one of the least effective methods of contraception. As a matter of fact people using the method have a name—parents.

However, if a woman has a regular menstrual cycle, there are benefits to this method. The time of ovulation is established by charting changes in your body temperature. Take your temperature at the same time each morning, just before rising. Record your temperature each day during the entire cycle. When ovulation begins, a woman's body temperature drops slightly, followed by a rise of about 0.5°F. over 24 to 72 hours. Theoretically intercourse should be avoided for two days prior to ovulation, the day of ovulation, and one day after ovulation. However, there are many variables affecting body temperature. For instance, your temperature normally varies throughout the day. On the other hand, if you have a cold or flu, you may have a change of temperature having nothing to do with ovulation. If you decide to use this method, be sure you know everything about the Rhythm Method before you start. Ask questions of your doctor and pharmacist. Don't rely on the experience of a friend; people are different, and if you don't get all the facts, you may be asking that same friend to babysit for you from time to time.

OVULATION METHOD

The Ovulation Method is a method of natural family planning that enables a woman to determine the fertile and infertile times of her menstrual cycle. A woman or couple is then able to make decisions to avoid or achieve pregnancy based on the presence of mucus or dryness at the opening of the vagina. The Ovulation Method not only is a mode of family planning, but also gives the woman invaluable insights into the events which occur during her menstrual cycle. It is important to recognize the fact that fertility is dependent on both the male and female; however, in this book only the woman's fertility is discussed.

The Ovulation Method gives a woman an understanding of her body. For example, she can learn to distinguish whether her observations of the vagina reveal a normal sequence of events or a possible disease process. Therefore, a woman using this method provides herself with a useful reproductive-health screening tool.

The Ovulation Method consists of checking for discharge at the opening of the vagina. If a discharge is present, she needs to record its consistency, color, and sensation and to note any changes which may occur in the discharge from one day to the next.

The menstrual cycle begins with the menstrual flow. Following the flow is usually a period of days that are free of vaginal discharge. Then begins a discharge of thick, sticky or tacky, and cloudy mucus. This discharge changes over a period of days to become clear, stretchy, and/or lubricative. This clear mucus is known as "peak-like" mucus. The last day of clear mucous discharge is called the "peak." Following the peak there is a dramatic change in the mucus, due to the drop in estrogen levels and the increase of progesterone which occurs after ovulation. The remaining days of the menstrual cycle are usually days in which no vaginal discharge appears.

There are many health benefits to women using the Ovulation Method. Some women have been able to determine, and therefore secure treatment for, VAGINAL INFECTIONS and CERVICITIS. Also, she can become familiar with the length of her menstrual cycle and the duration and amount of menstrual flow. Since the occurrence of menstrual periods follows ovulation by an average of fourteen days, a woman using the Ovulation Method learns to expect her period in twelve to sixteen days after her peak. Also, she is able to recognize the effects of illness and stress on her menstrual cycle.

A couple can use the Ovulation Method to avoid or to achieve pregnancy. If they wish to avoid pregnancy they should not have genital contact on fertile days. If they wish to achieve pregnancy they will have intercourse on fertile days, the best time being on the days of peak-like mucus. The effects of drugs, nutrition, stress, and light on the menstrual cycle are areas of research to which the Ovulation Method lends itself and which are currently being investigated.

In conclusion, the Ovulation Method is an invaluable health tool as well as an effective natural family planning method. It is useful during a woman's entire fertile years, preceding menarche and through menopause. Learning the Ovulation Method requires frequent follow-up visits with a trained instructor during the early stages. Ongoing, update follow-ups are recommended to reinforce and re-evaluate the woman's or the couple's understanding of the technique.

10
COSMETICS

One area of the typical drugstore dedicated entirely to women is the COSMETICS counter. Of course this area has helped a lot of men out of trouble, as a place to buy that last-minute birthday or anniversary gift.

Nowadays there are more cosmetics on the shelves than you can imagine, with each company making competing claims. The biggest problem is pronouncing the names of some of these products, because they don't sound like they're spelled.

Let's face it: Looking good adds a dimension of confidence and ease that you don't have when your hair is all wrong, your face is broken out, and your body is out of shape. One of the most important beauty assets a young woman can have is healthy, glowing skin, from head to toe. Today's make-up look is lighter and more transparent.

Although most cosmetics on the market today are hypo-allergenic (which means they are low in allergens), ALLERGIC REACTIONS and IRRITANT REACTIONS still do occur. Irritant reactions commonly occur the first time a woman comes in contact with a particular cosmetic, while allergic reactions generally develop after continued use.

Whether you use liquid, pressed-powder, or solid-cake

cosmetics, you may develop a reaction if you use it too often or too heavily. Most cosmetics counters have a sales clerk who knows even more about these products than the pharmacist. Ask her advice about your cosmetics; the more you know the less likely you are to develop problems.

Some perfumes may react with the skin to form a new chemical that causes irritation, such as FORMALDEHYDE. Although one doesn't associate perfume with formaldehyde, the reaction sometimes occurs.

Reactions to soap, cosmetics, and other beauty aids can be a problem for any woman. But you *can* minimize their harmfulness and, if they do affect you, treat the symptoms successfully.

The first and most obvious step is avoidance of irritating or allergenic products. Second, do not do anything to further irritate an area that is already affected. And third, use cool water compresses on the affected area for five to ten minutes several times a day. You may even use one of the over-the-counter hydrocortisone creams or ointments such as CORTAID or CLEAR AID that are now available without a prescription.

Cosmetics other than perfumes, toilet waters, and the like deteriorate with age. The older the cosmetic, the more susceptible it is to bacteria and the more likely you are to get a bacteria-caused reaction. Don't buy more than you can use in six months. Keeping make-up in the refrigerator will slow its deterioration.

Also remember that, no matter what cosmetic you use, it is designed for use on healthy skin. You are asking for trouble if you apply any beauty aid to an area that is already irritated. As always, if the problem persists for an abnormal length of time, see your doctor.

The key to good skin is a balanced diet. Adequate vitamins absorbed from a proper diet are essential to having good skin. Some cosmetics contain VITAMIN E OIL, and some people simply apply the oil inside a vitamin E capsule to the skin to promote healthy skin. Unfortunately vitamin E sometimes causes allergic reactions or acne. Too much

VITAMIN A may cause the skin, especially the soles of the feet and the palms of the hands, to yellow and lead to uncomfortable dryness. The point is that too many vitamins, as well as too few, can have undesirable side effects.

Women are finding more and newer products at the cosmetic counter. Traditional fingernail polish removers are side-by-side with polish-removing gels, in which you simply place your fingers—the polish comes off in a few minutes. The regular nail polish removers are still available and probably work faster.

There are also a variety of ways for removing make-up. Soap-and-water treatment is probably still the most common. But that sometimes leaves the skin dried out, so it might be to your advantage to apply a cream moisturizer to your face after washing it. And of course there is the old stand-by, cold cream. Rub it all over your face, then wipe it away after a few minutes with a tissue. This way of removing make-up does have the advantage of keeping your skin moist. Another way is to use the cleansing pads that are pre-moistened with mineral oil. While you wipe away the make-up, the mineral oil keeps the skin soft and lubricated. These products may cost a little bit more but it sure takes the fuss and mess out of removing make-up. Next time you are near the cosmetic counter take a look at what is available. You will probably be surprised—there's always something new.

11

DENTAL PRODUCTS

Although there are more than 100,000 dentists in the United States, dental disease is a very common health problem. The problem is that dental care is not considered a major health priority; usually we only go to a dentist in the event of an emergency, after the damage has been done. Teeth are made to last a lifetime provided proper care is taken. Some pharmacies carry almost every dental product on the market, others have a rather limited selection. Dentists and patients appreciate a wide selection of products, but you may need guidance in making your choice.

TOOTHBRUSHES

Deciding among all the different types of toothbrushes that are available is often a source of confusion—let alone trying to find the color that would be best in your bathroom, overnight case, or that matches your bathrobe. The important thing is to chose a toothbrush that will do a good job of cleaning your teeth. Most dentists recommend a soft to medium nylon bristle. Brushing with too-hard bristles irritates the gum line and may cause bleeding, thereby keeping you from brushing thoroughly. Your toothbrush needs to be replaced every two months. It should be small, in order to reach all tooth surfaces and to fit in the rear of the mouth and on the tongue side of the teeth. Some people complain of gagging when brushing; in that case try using a child's size toothbrush.

The Council on Dental Materials has so far not found that using a powered toothbrush produces better results than manual brushing. Therefore, use whatever one helps you to brush continuously and effectively. In some cases, as with small children and patients suffering from diseases (including multiple sclerosis or cerebral palsy), the powered toothbrush makes brushing the teeth much easier; in the case of children, the novelty may make it more interesting. Also, it should be pointed out that brushing cannot remove plaque. A trip to the dentist is necessary for that. But no matter how good a toothbrush you select, it will only do half the job unless you use a good toothpaste right along with it.

TOOTHPASTE

Toothpastes are used with a toothbrush to clean the teeth. They are available in pastes, powders, and gels. They contain abrasives, flavoring, and foaming agents. These products help remove stains and plaque. If they taste good they encourage you to brush more often. The best toothpaste is one with the greatest amount of stain remover and the least amount of abrasiveness. Some of the toothpastes, as well as some of the tooth powders, that are intended to remove stains more effectively and whiten or brighten the teeth are highly abrasive and should not be used regularly. Some toothpastes contain fluoride, and when used regularly can help reduce the incidence of cavities. However, some dentists feel that fluoride toothpastes are more effective in children than in adults. Because of the chemicals that build up on the teeth of an adult, it is hard for the fluoride to penetrate through that barrier and protect the teeth. People often are confused about which toothpaste to buy. A good rule of thumb is to look at the package and see if it has been accepted by the American Dental Association. The ones that have been accepted have the least amount of abrasiveness, as well as the right amount of fluoride to adequately protect the teeth. Toothpastes that have been accepted by the Council on Dental Therapeutics are AIM, CREST, AQUAFRESH, COLGATE MFP, and MACLEANS. People with sensitive teeth should use a toothpaste for sensitive teeth, such as PROTECT, SENSODYNE, and THERMODENT.

DENTAL FLOSS AND TAPE

Dental floss is essential for removing plaque and debris in areas your toothbrush cannot reach. The crevices between the teeth and along the gum line attract bacteria, which can get to the tooth and destroy it. When using dental floss, use a sawing motion to move it between the teeth. Avoid forcing it down between the teeth, which may result in an injury to the gum. Dental floss is available in waxed and unwaxed varieties. Most dentists recommend the unwaxed floss, because the waxed floss sometimes leaves deposits of wax on the tooth. These in turn may cause plaque to stick to it and remain on the tooth. Waxed floss is usually used by people with tightly spaced teeth, because it moves more easily between the teeth. Dental tape or ribbon is another form available. There is no functional difference between floss, ribbon, or tape; choice is simply a matter of personal preference.

DISCLOSING AGENTS

A new type of dental product now available in most drugstores is a *disclosing agent*. It is available in either liquid or tablet form. These products are very useful in teaching children, as well as adults, to brush their teeth properly. Disclosing agents such as **RED COTE** contain a red dye. All you do is to chew one of the tablets, or swish a few drops of the liquid around your mouth just before brushing. Both forms stain or color the plaque and debris on the teeth; you then simply brush off all the red color. By doing this every night for a week or two, you will develop a fairly effective method for brushing your teeth correctly. Often we think we brush our teeth properly when in fact we only do half the job. If you want to train your children as well as yourself to brush teeth properly, disclosing agents can help—it is like having someone show you the proper technique. The red dye in these products is **FD** and **C RED #3,** which is perfectly safe and suitable for home use.

DENTURES

People who have not taken care of their teeth, or who have lost them through gum disease or an accident of some sort, can be fitted for dentures. Not surprisingly, there are now just about as many different products for use with dentures as for natural teeth.

DENTURE ADHESIVES

For example, there are just about as many adhesives to keep your dentures in place as there are toothpastes. Some of them are paste, others are powder. Some of the well-known denture adhesive brands are **CORECA POWDER, EFFERGRIP powder** and **cream, FASTEETH, FIXODENT, ORAFIX, POLI-GRIP,** and **WERNET'S cream** and **powder.** Be careful when using these products. Sometimes people who continually use adhesives cannot tell if their dentures are out of alignment and need an adjustment. If your dentures do get out of alignment, they put pressure on various areas of the gum, creating painful sores and perhaps causing damage to the mouth itself. Prolonged use of adhesives, if dentures are not cleaned regularly, may stimulate the growth of bacteria, causing bad breath and infections in the mouth. Therefore, before using the adhesive products, be sure to cleanse the dentures thoroughly. If you do notice any irritation of the gum or uncomfortable pressure, check with your dentist. You may be able to prevent a lot of problems before they get started.

DENTURE CLEANSERS

To avoid permanent staining and bad breath, you must brush your dentures at least once daily: Even though you don't have teeth of your own, you still can't get away with not brushing. But be careful not to brush too hard with an abrasive material. Any denture cleansers on the market are good to use, because they are compatible with the material your dentures are made from. Toilet soap and baking soda are also suitable cleansers for dentures, although they probably are not as effective as some of the prepared cleansers you can buy. No matter what denture cleanser you use, it is important to rinse the dentures thoroughly before placing them in your mouth. (Since some of these cleansing agents are corrosive, keep them well out of the reach of children. Every year there are a number of accidental poisonings as a result of kids eating these and other over-the-counter products.) Sometimes soaking your dentures in undiluted white vinegar will remove stubborn stains. Again, be sure to rinse them thoroughly before putting them back in your mouth.

SONIC AND ULTRASONIC DENTURE CLEANERS

Sonic and ultrasonic denture-cleaning devices are relatively new products. They are electric. When you plug them in, they produce a current in the water, which, as it passes over the dentures, removes food particles and debris. Such a product makes a thoughtful gift, especially for the elderly, who have trouble cleaning their dentures. There are three distinct kinds to choose from. The *ultrasonic* is the most effective, the *magnetic stirrers* second in effectiveness, and the *vibrator* least effective. If you need help in selecting the product ask your pharmacist or, better yet, call your dentist and see what he recommends.

RELINERS AND REPAIR KITS

Dentures that don't fit properly may simply need a slight adjustment. However, poor fit may also indicate a change in the bone structure of your mouth. You should see your dentist. You may think that using a reliner on your denture will solve the problem. Wrong! These products can actually be dangerous, especially if used over a long period of time. They may change the shape of your denture or make it fit too tightly. This causes additional pressure on the gums and bone, as well as irritating the tongue and cheeks, causing sores that could lead to cancerous lesions. It would be best if these products were simply banned, or made available only by a prescription from a dentist.

Occasionally people drop their dentures and break them. You may be tempted to show that you are a good craftsman by gluing yours back together, or using one of the denture repair kits. *Do not do it yourself.* If you do not line up the denture exactly, it will once again put additional pressure on the gums, causing the same problems that the denture reliners cause. As a matter of fact, the F.D.A. considers reliners and repair kits unsafe. Unfortunately, they are still on the market, and as long as there is a demand for them, you'll find them in drugstores along with the other dental products.

TOOTHACHE DROPS

Toothache drops are an old stand-by for a toothache. It always seems that toothaches develop on weekends, or in the evening when the dentist is not in his office. So you run out and buy one of the toothache products available at the drug store. These products contain either BENZOCAINE or EUGENOL (the active ingredient in OIL OF CLOVES), which produces a local anesthetic action on the tooth or gum. Unfortunately, these products are not very effective and may sometimes injure the tooth further. Aspirin, as well as other over-the-counter pain relievers, may be useful for relieving the pain temporarily. However, under no circumstances should these products be applied directly to the teeth or gums. Aspirin will burn the tissue surrounding the tooth, as well as the tongue, causing sores that can take a long time to heal. It can also cause further damage to the tooth. Remember that toothache is a local problem that should be treated locally by a dentist. Pain relievers treat only the symptom and not the cause.

So have a periodic check-up with your dentist, because more Americans lack dental care than have it. Those who take the proper preventative steps will have the fewest problems.

There are other products available in the drugstore such as an electric tooth buffer, to help you clean your teeth more easily. A tooth buffer is similar to what the dentist uses to clean your teeth. It consists of a handle with a round rubber end. When you plug it in, the rubber tip spins and is used to buff or polish the teeth. I would like to point out, however, that even though it resembles the one your dentist uses on your teeth, he has a lot more experience in using it. If used improperly, a tooth buffer can cause an injury to the tooth or gum.

Another product that has gained in popularity is the WATER-PIK. It squirts a pulsating stream of water to remove food particles and prevent the formation of bacteria between the teeth, which may otherwise cause the loss of teeth due to gum disease. Some claim that this product work better than flossing. However, if you point the stream directly at the gum, it may cause the gum to pull away from the tooth. You can adjust the force of water, so make sure it is neither too strong nor too weak to really clean between the teeth and at the gum line. If you are considering buying one, you might want to talk it over with your pharmacist, or with your dentist, to make sure that you know not only all the facts about the product but also how to use it properly.

12

DEODORANTS

Now here's a topic that's really the "pits": underarm deodorants. Needless to say, advertisers have a field day promoting these products. For example, when a certain manufacturer came out with "five-day" deodorant pads, I wonder how many people walked around for five days with pads stuck under their arms? And how many thought they only had to use them every five days? By the fifth day they probably had very few friends. Deodorants are available in many different shapes and forms as well as in a wide range of fragrances. Deodorants are odor-maskers, while anti-perspirants prevent perspiration. Since body odor occurs when we sweat (bacteria grows in such a warm, moist environment, causing odor), the best thing to use is an anti-perspirant. These products are rubbed or sprayed under the arms. They irritate the sweat glands, causing them to swell and block the pores, thereby preventing sweat from being secreted by the sweat glands. Though it sounds simple, it may not seem so when you arrive at the drugstore to buy them and find rows and rows of different brands. Which one to pick? What offers the best bargain? Which one will do the best job for you? Some deodorants, usually those in stick form, are nothing more than a fragrance to mask body odor.

Examples are MENNEN SPEED STICK, OLD SPICE, CHAZ, JOVAN, BRITISH STERLING, BRUT, and ENGLISH LEATHER. Other products actually contain ingredients to prevent body odor.

ZIRCONIUM is an ingredient found in many of the liquid roll-on deodorants and some stick deodorants, for example SOFT AND DRY, SECRET, DRY IDEA, and DIAL. That is why deodorants usually contain zirconium along with another ingredient to stop wetness (such as ALUMINUM CHLOROHYDRATE). It has antiseptic properties and works by killing bacteria. By killing the bacteria, you prevent body odor. Avoid leaving a soapy residue on the skin after bathing, because it will react with zirconium, making it ineffective. Be sure that your skin is rinsed thoroughly and dried. Some people have told me that they use a mixture of SODIUM BICARBONATE (baking soda) and their favorite talcum powder, which they sprinkle or rub under their arms. They say it works and is very inexpensive to use. I suppose if a box of baking soda placed in the sink drain and in ice boxes absorbs odor it ought to work under your arms. However, this would probably only work if your problem wasn't too bad.

Anti-perspirants are not only the most effective but also the most commonly available preparations for preventing body odor. Usually they contain ALUMINUM CHLORIDE or ALUMINUM CHLOROHYDRATE.

ALUMINUM CHLORIDE is probably one of the most effective single ingredients to prevent perspiration. But aluminum chloride has its side effects. For example, when aluminum chloride comes into contact with wet skin, it causes stinging, irritation, and burning. It may fade or rot clothing. As a matter of fact nowadays there are hardly any deodorants with aluminum chloride in them. Most manufacturers are using ALUMINUM CHLOROHYDRATE in place of it. ALUMINUM CHLOROHYDRATE is a more refined version of aluminum chloride. It works the same way as aluminum chloride but creates fewer problems. Products that use this more refined ingredient usually have the names "dry," "dry formula," "extra dry," and "super dry." But don't go by the label alone. Pick up the product and read the ingredients yourself. Make sure it says aluminum chlorohydrate. This ingredient is available in sprays, roll-ons, and sticks. Among others, aluminum chlorohydrate is found in MITCHUM, TICKLE, MUM, TUSSY, RIGHT GUARD, SURE, and BAN.

If you use aerosol sprays, try not to inhale them; they could be harmful. Since one normally sprays deodorant in a bathroom where the ventilation is minimal, a good rule of thumb is that if you can smell the spray, you are certainly breathing it in. If you notice any sort of rash or irritation of the area where you apply your deodorant, stop using that particular kind. Some people are more sensitive than others to certain ingredients. If the rash is at all uncomfortable, you might want to apply one of the over-the-counter HYDRO-CORTISONE creams like CORTAID for a couple of days to help clear up the irritation. And be sure not to use another product with the same ingredient. There might be other ingredients in the deodorant that could irritate your skin, so be sure to check the ingredients listed on the container and through the process of elimination you might find the one causing your problem.

An important thing to think about when you buy a deoderant is what you want the product to do. Since these products all contain the same active ingredient, it is difficult to know how any one can be better than another. Keep that in mind and buy the cheapest one.

13

DIARRHEA

A condition that is the source of much humor is no joking matter for the person who has it. Diarrhea can be caused by a variety of different agents, such as a virus, drugs of various sorts, and certain foods. Diarrhea in infants and young children is common. Its incidence is often attributed to a viral infection of the intestinal tract.

Viral diarrhea usually develops rapidly without any warning signals, lasts about one to two days, and produces a low-grade fever. However, diarrhea in small children can be dangerous. The loss of water and salts in a short period of time may cause severe dehydration, which could develop into serious complications resulting in circulatory collapse and kidney failure.

The characteristics of the stool can be helpful in determining the cause of diarrhea. For example, undigested food particles in the stool indicate small-intestine irritation. Black, tarry stool can mean upper intestinal bleeding or bleeding from the stomach. Red stool may indicate large-intestine bleeding, or perhaps simply eating a food containing a red dye, such as beets. At this point it would be a good idea to check with your doctor before using over-the-counter products.

Diarrhea is a symptom of a problem; therefore, treatment should be aimed at the problem causing the diarrhea and not just at stopping the mad dashes to the bathroom, unpleasant though these may be.

ABSORBENTS

ABSORBENTS are the type of ingredient most frequently found in over-the-counter anti-diarrhea products such as KAOLIN, PECTIN, and BISMUTH SUBSALICYLATE. They work by absorbing nutrients, toxins, and bacteria from the intestinal tract. Because they are generally taken in large doses, most of them are flavored to taste good. Absorbents are generally used in the treatment of minor diarrhea, because they are safe and have the ability to absorb digested materials as well as bacteria and other irritating matter when taken orally. These products are not themselves absorbed. They act like a sponge in the intestines, and they sometimes cause constipation.

However, people using an absorbent diarrhea product should be careful if they are taking any other type of medicine, because it may interfere with the body's ability to absorb the medicine properly. Before buying this or any product, it would be wise to talk it over with your pharmacist first.

Absorbents are usually taken after each loose bowel movement until the diarrhea is controlled. Some of the products that fall into this class are: KAOPECTATE, KAOPECTATE CONCENTRATE, and PEPTO-BISMOL liquid and tablets.

Other products used to treat diarrhea contain additional ingredients, such as the BELLADONNA ALKALOIDS found in a product like DONNAGEL. When diarrhea is due to increased intestinal activity, this product will slow it down. Such products should be used on children only with the consent of your doctor, and people who have glaucoma or pressure in the eyes should avoid them. If you do take them and notice a blurring of vision, rapid pulse, or dizziness, stop. These products are not intended for long use. If you develop dryness of the mouth, decrease the dose you are taking.

Years ago PAREGORIC was used to treat diarrhea. Aside from the horrible taste, it worked well to stop diarrhea. Paregoric contains an opium derivative which works directly on the small intestine and colon to slow them down, thereby slowing the passage of intestinal contents as well. This in turn causes us to reabsorb water and salts into the intestines and stops diarrhea.

Nowadays paregoric is available only on a doctor's prescription. Because of its narcotic content, people began to abuse the drug. Some people became hooked on it and went from drugstore to drugstore to buy bottles of it. Pharmacists could only sell a maximum of two ounces in a 48-hour period to a single individual, so at the time of the sale each person signed his or her name and address in a record book.

Although paregoric became a prescription drug, it is still available without a prescription in combination products— that is in products that contain paregoric along with other anti-diarrheals, such as AMOGEL, DONNAGEL-PG, PARE-LIXIR, PAREPECTOLIN, and PABIZOL WITH PAREGORIC.

If you decide to use a paregoric-containing preparation, remember that you won't find it on the shelf in the drugstore. You still must sign a register for these products, and you will have to ask the pharmacist for it, because they usually keep it behind the prescription counter.

Sometimes people develop diarrhea when they take certain kinds of prescription medicines, such as ANTIBIOTICS. Since these are made to kill bacteria, they may kill the good bacteria in our stomach and intestines that are responsible for proper intestinal and bowel functions, resulting in diarrhea. There are some products that restore normal intestinal bacteria, such as BACID capsules and LACTINEX tablets and granules, that have been destroyed by antibiotics.

If you don't have any of these products at home, it also sometimes helps to drink buttermilk. Be sure first that you can drink it while taking the antibiotic, since milk can interact with the TETRACYCLINE antibiotics. Drink it one hour before or two hours after a dose of your medicine.

Although people joke about diarrhea, it can cause serious problems. If we lose too much fluid, we become dehydrated. This is especially dangerous in children, because it happens so fast. If your child has diarrhea, keep a close eye on him or her. It might help to take the temperature often, to make sure it is not getting too high from the loss of fluids. If the child develops a fever, call your doctor immediately, and have the patient drink plenty of fluids. If you notice blood, or if the stool becomes very slimy, call your doctor; diarrhea may not be your only problem.

14
DIET AIDS

Obesity is defined as a condition in which actual body weight is more than 20 percent higher than the ideal weight. A rule of thumb for determining your ideal weight is

- Men five feet tall should weigh 106 pounds, with six additional pounds for every inch over five feet. If you are five feet, eight inches tall, ideally you would weigh 154 pounds.
- Women five feet tall should weigh 100 pounds, with an additional five pounds for every inch over five feet.

Based on this definition, it is estimated that 35 percent of Americans of all ages are obese, as is more than 50 percent of the adult population. People from every social and economic group are concerned about being overweight—especially women. But despite the risks, most of us continue to overeat. The principal culprit in making us overweight is an excess of calories, of which every food contains a certain number.

A calorie is a measurement of the energy in foods, but

that is only half the story. The energy your body uses each day is also measured in calories. The whole idea of weight control is that the number of calories you take in each day should just about equal the number of calories you use. But what happens to the calories you don't use? Under the skin are millions of tiny cells. Extra food calories are converted in our bodies to a fatty substance and stored inside these cells. It may not sound like much, but an excess of even 150 calories adds up. Repeated calorie surpluses cause the fat cells to enlarge, and 150-calorie surplus every day for one year would end up as fifteen pounds of fat.

We must learn to think in terms of how people become overweight in the first place. Obesity is much easier to prevent than it is to cure. We always say that a fat baby is a healthy baby, but in fact parents often overfeed their children. Infancy and childhood are the times in our lives when fat cells are being formed. Overfeeding can cause excess fat cells to develop; these remain in the body throughout life, making it forever hard for that child to lose weight as he or she grows up.

Along with fat cells, habits and attitudes are also being formed in early life. Many parents use food as a bribe for good behavior, so that the child gets the idea that food is a reward. This attitude may carry over into later life. As an adult, every time the person feels frustrated, discouraged, or depressed he stuffs himself with food to feel better. Some parents instill in their children the idea that they have to eat everything on their plates, whether they want it or not, and then afterwards reward them with sweets such as ice cream.

Eating habits are very hard to change. That is why it is best to convey good eating habits to children when they are young. The older one gets the harder it is to change them.

American men and women tend to add both pounds and inches as the years go by. As you become less active, your metabolism slows down, although your eating habits may remain unchanged. Consequently, over-the-counter diet aids have become a multimillion-dollar industry. Most of

the newer products contain an ingredient called PHENYL-
PROPANOLAMINE or PPA.

PHENYLPROPANOLAMINE (PPA)

Chemically related to EPHEDRINE and AMPHETAMINE,
PPA is also found in many of the cold and sinus preparations
as a decongestant. It does stimulate the central nervous system to some degree. However, experts say that the stimulation is not enough to suppress the appetite. Manufacturers
continue to promote products such as DIETAC and DEXA-
TRIM, and there are people who swear by these products
because they used them and actually lost weight. That may
be more a psychological result than anything else. In one
double-blind test, subjects who took a placebo (sugar pills)
and those who took a capsule with phenylpropanolamine
showed very little difference in weight loss. Perhaps someone ought to make a product that doesn't contain anything
at all; it will probably work very well.

PHENYLPROPANOLAMINE does have side effects, especially if you exceed the recommended dose. Nervousness,
restlessness, insomnia, headache, and nausea, as well as
increase in blood pressure, have been reported by people
taking these products. There have also been reports of PPA
causing palpitations. If you suffer from high blood pressure
to begin with, be sure to check with a doctor who knows
your medical background. Chances are that if he has prescribed medication for you to keep your blood pressure
under control, he will not want you to use these products.
Some people suffering from arthritis take a prescription
drug called INDOCIN. When Indocin is combined with
phenylpropanolamine, it sometimes causes a hypertensive
crisis—that is, a marked increase in blood pressure to a dangerous level. Some over-the-counter products contain CAF-
FEINE along with the PHENYLPROPANOLAMINE. Both
ingredients affect the heart and blood vessels, and in combination are more likely to result in side effects.

Be sure to check with your doctor before taking any of these products. If you have any questions about the ingredients, don't rely on the testimony of a friend who used the product. Ask your pharmacist to help you decide which product is safe for you to use.

BULK-PRODUCING DIET AIDS

These diet aids contain ingredients such as METHYLCELLULOSE, CARBOXYMETHYLCELLULOSE, PSYLLIUM, AGAR, and KARAYA GUM, which work by absorbing water. Water absorption causes them to swell, producing a sense of fullness, which in turn reduces the desire to eat. The problem is that these products have been shown to leave the stomach in about thirty minutes. When they reach the intestine they stimulate bowel movement. Thus, one is taking a product that reduces hunger for about 30 minutes, but also creates a laxative effect. The benefit of these diet aids is that they can help cut down on the intake of calories, but they are no more effective than a low-calorie diet alone. If you are one of those people who simply can't stick to a diet, these products may help to some degree. If you do decide to use one of these products, such as AYDS candy, SLIM-LINE candy, or MELOZETS wafers, be sure to drink plenty of water with it. If your doctor has prescribed a medicine for your stomach or to slow down your intestinal movements, you could cause intestinal blockage if you combine it with a bulk-producing diet aid.

BENZOCAINE

When we hear the word BENZOCAINE, we usually think of something to rub on the skin to deaden it. But some products containing benzocaine are taken orally. Many of them are in the form of hard candy. The idea is to numb the inside of your mouth, thereby reducing the desire to eat, especially if you are a constant snacker. People chew or suck one of these candy products when they have the urge to eat. This keeps the mouth active, and the products do work to some degree. However, most of the products are in capsule and tablet form and the drug itself is swallowed before it comes into contact with the mouth, making it less effective. Benzocaine causes allergic reactions in some people.

LOW-CALORIE BALANCED FOODS

Canned diet products are used as substitutes for the usual diet. These products are available in powders, liquids, and granules, as well as cookies and soups. Dietary foods are low in SODIUM. Therefore weight loss in the first two weeks is probably caused by water loss from the tissues in the body. However, the long-term benefits of these products are questionable. If you use the liquid form of food substitutes but don't really care for the taste, try chilling it. It will taste a lot better.

ARTIFICIAL SWEETENERS

Sugar overuse is common. It is also responsible for adding more than a large number of empty calories to the diet. A sugar substitute, SACCHARIN, provides no calories and may aid calorie reduction for certain people. Saccharin is about 400 times sweeter than sugar, but has a bitter taste for some people. Nevertheless, it is the most popular artificial sweetener, especially since the use of cyclamates was discontinued. In 1972, bladder tumors were discovered in rats that were fed saccharin. The F.D.A. then removed saccharin from the list of food additives generally recognized as safe. Saccharin is presently permitted in products labeled specifically as diet foods or beverages. The problem caused quite a bit of controversy in the medical profession, as well as a lot of confusion on the part of the public. Pregnant women are advised *not* to use saccharin during their pregnancy. As of June 1978, pharmacies carrying saccharin-containing over-the-counter products are required to display posters containing a warning that saccharin has been determined to cause cancer in laboratory animals.

As alternatives to SACCHARIN, there are two other sugar substitutes. One of them is SORBITAL, and the other is XYLI-TOL. These products are not as sweet as saccharin, but they do have advantages. Neither of these products causes tooth decay, and some products containing XYLITOL have a more pleasant taste than those containing saccharin. There is some evidence that xylitol is implicated in the development of bladder tumors in mice, so its use is on the decline. Many of the dietetic gums and candies contain sorbital and MAN-NATAL as sweetening agents. But these ingredients can have a laxative effect, especially in children. Eating a whole package of mints can cause cramps and diarrhea. Parents often dismiss it by thinking it is just "something they ate." You are right there, Mom! If you notice that your child develops intestinal distress every time he or she has a sugarless mint or gum, reward him or her in another way.

A new sweetener called ASPARTAME has recently been approved by the Food and Drug Administration. It is marketed under the trade name EQUAL. It is an alternative to SACCHARIN, which the F.D.A. still considers to be unsafe. Aspartame is available in tablets and powder packets. It has also been approved for manufacturers' use in instant powdered drinks, cereals, and sugarless gums. The Searle Company will apply shortly for permission to use it in diet sodas.

One packet of EQUAL (4 calories) is equivalent in sweetness to two teaspoons of sugar (36 calories). It also doesn't have the bitter aftertaste that saccharin has.

Aspartame is made by combining amino acids, the building blocks of protein, like those found naturally in meats and cheese. Therefore this product is broken down more rapidly than saccharin, and eliminated from the body. Since the approval of aspartame there has been a lot of controversy over the safety of this product. A question of whether it may cause brain damage has been raised, and some doctors feel that more animal tests for cancer should be done on the product. But the F.D.A. has said that, judging by available test data, these are unreasonable fears.

GROUP THERAPY

Group therapy has been proven very effective in treating obesity. Groups such as TOPS (Take Off Pounds Sensibly) and Weight Watchers have successful treatment records for obesity. Group pressure and support has proven to be a good deterrent to overeating for many persons. Also, eating more slowly causes you to feel satisfied more quickly; therefore you eat less. These organizations have a lot of useful suggestions, as well as special weight reduction programs that can help you lose weight. They teach you how to eat for the rest of your life.

No matter what type of action you take to fight the battle of the bulge, remember that unless you change your dietary habits you will gain back any weight you lose. And no matter what type of over-the-counter products you decide to use, it will never take the place of a good diet and exercise.

15

DRY SKIN

For some people dry or chapped skin is an allergic condition that flares up now and then, usually with the change in seasons. Whatever the reason for dry skin, it is annoying and uncomfortable because of the constant itching and, in some cases, pain and inflammation. Dry skin is also more susceptible to bacterial infections than normal skin.

Dry skin is characterized by roughness, flaking, and tightness. As the word "dry" implies, dry skin results from a loss of moisture. The best way to treat dry skin is to replace the water that has been lost. However, adding water to the skin is useless unless the skin can retain it. If wet skin is not covered immediately with a substance like VASELINE or plastic, it will become dehydrated again quickly.

There are shelves and shelves of products to treat dry skin to be found in the drugstore. Nevertheless, they all fall into two basic types: products to lubricate the skin and products to moisturize the skin.

LUBRICATING LOTIONS

These products are mainly intended to lubricate the skin, causing it to feel smooth. In other words they are a strictly psychological approach to dry skin. Even though the skin feels smooth, it may not be back to normal. Most of the lubricating products are cosmetic: They are pretty effective at correcting the dry skin condition, but they don't get to the root of the problem of why you had dry skin to begin with. Lubricating lotions contain ingredients like mineral oil, water, and lanolin and are found in products like LUBRI-DERM lotion and KERI lotion.

MOISTURIZING LOTIONS AND CREAMS

These products contain ingredients to replace the moisture your skin has lost. Some lotions contain GLYCERIN to treat dry skin; products such as CORN HUSKERS and GLYC-ERIN AND ROSE WATER are very good at moisturizing the skin. Glycerin acts as a "magnet" to draw water from the atmosphere, holding it until the skin needs more water. Although lotions containing glycerin are somewhat effective in treating dry skin, glycerin does not penetrate the skin too well, and there must be enough water in the air for the glycerin to draw it to the skin. And if there were a lot of moisture in the air, one probably wouldn't have the dry skin condition to begin with. Most of the products that you can buy contain only 50 percent glycerin. You can make your own glycerin lotion at home by mixing glycerin with an equal part water. Other products used to treat dry skin are lotions made of VEGETABLE or MINERAL OIL. Oils cause the skin to become more flexible; they also form a barrier over the skin to keep the skin from losing water. However, mineral oil products are absorbed by the skin more effectually than vegetable oil.

No one likes to apply oil directly to his or her skin because it feels greasy. However, oils, found in products such as LUBATH and ALPHA KERI, may be put into the bath water to help moisturize dry skin. These do help lubricate the skin, and they may be applied directly to the skin if you so choose. If you decide to use a bath oil, take some precaution such as putting a towel in the bottom of the bathtub; oily water can cause the bathtub to become extremely slippery and the towel will prevent you from falling. Don't use a bath mat, because it will become as slippery as the tub itself.

Many companies combine OIL with WATER, resulting in a cloudy mixture, or lotion. Other ingredients are added to hold it in a lotion form. Most of the products found in the drugstore to treat dry skin are lotions containing oil and water: VASELINE INTENSIVE CARE, KERI LOTION, JERGENS—the list is endless. The mineral-oil-and-water products might be a little better to use, because they are absorbed into the skin better. Using a water-and-oil lotion may help to relieve itching because of the cooling effect as the water evaporates from the skin surface. Most of these products do not produce a greasy, oily feeling on the skin.

VITAMIN A is useful in treating some skin conditions. As a matter of fact, one of the effects of vitamin A in the diet is to promote the growth of healthy skin. Dermatologists have been using it for years, along with other treatments. There are skin lotions that contain vitamin A, as well as VITAMIN E and VITAMIN D. But since absorption through the skin is poor, using these vitamins topically has very little effect on a dry skin condition. Dermatologists usually use vitamin A orally to treat some cases of acne. But since vitamin A can be stored in the body, it's best you take it under a doctor's supervision so he can watch out for any unusual side effects.

ALOE VERA

Many of the newer lotions on the market contain the juice of a plant that people may have in their homes, and which is called an aloe plant. The leaves of the plant are thick and fleshy and contain a jellylike substance called ALOE VERA GEL. Manufacturers are now using this natural moisturizer in various skin care products. It is an excellent nutrient for the skin, because it contains proteins, vitamins, and minerals, and helps remove dead skin and stimulate the growth of new skin. If you have used various lotions to treat your dry skin but feel that you haven't gotten results, you may want to try a product that contains aloe.

COSMETICS AND SKIN

The perfumes that are in some cosmetics may cause skin problems. In spite of their good smell, when they come into contact with the skin, they may break down into other compounds that cause irritation to the skin. Reaction to soap, cosmetics, and other beauty aids can be a problem for anyone. Even though most cosmetics today are hypoallergenic (that is, they are less likely to cause an allergic reaction) some people still develop very irritating reactions. These reactions usually occur the first time you come into contact with a cosmetic. Often they are caused by using the product incorrectly—too often or too heavily, for example. The product then damages the skin where it is applied. If this occurs, the first and most obvious step is to avoid the product. You may want to pick up a HYDROCORTISONE cream or lotion to apply to the irritated area. Hydrocortisone topical products are now available without a prescription, under the names of CORTAID, WELLCORTIN, and many others. Hydrocortisone products provide comfort and decrease the danger of infection from scratching. Hydrocortisone creams and lotions can be used for the temporary relief of ITCHING and RASHES due to ECZEMA and ALLERGIC REACTIONS due to poison ivy, poison oak, insect bites, jewelry, and other causes.

DISHPAN HANDS

The new term for dishpan hands is "housewife's eczema." This is a problem that affects a lot of women. It is a reaction caused by the ingredients in many household cleaners, such as dishwashing liquids, detergents, and various other cleaning products, when they come into contact with the skin. If you develop these skin problems after doing household chores, first wash your hands thoroughly and rinse them with cool water; while the hands are still wet apply any of the skin lotions we mentioned earlier, rub in well, then pat the hands dry with a clean towel. Also wear rubber gloves when doing the dishes or scrubbing the kitchen floor. By avoiding skin contact with these ingredients, the problems can be prevented. If you do develop very irritated skin on the hands, you might want to try one of the over-the-counter HYDROCORTISONE products. They work very well at relieving the ITCHING and INFLAMMATION due to ALLERGIC REACTIONS to various cleaners.

DIAPER RASH

There is one problem to which no infant is immune and that is DIAPER RASH. It usually shows up as a rash in the folds of the legs, but can spread over the entire diapered area. This condition is very painful for the child. It causes BURNING and ITCHING which can result in restlessness, irritability, and sleep interruption. If the rash spreads outside the diapered area, check with your doctor; it may be a sign of SKIN INFECTION or other problems. There are many different creams and lotions for the treatment of diaper rash. Some contain VITAMINS A and D. Vitamins A and D are very good for the skin when taken orally, but it is doubtful that they do much good when applied to the surface of the skin.

All creams for the treatment of diaper rash have one thing in common: They coat the skin to protect it from moisture and so prevent further irritation. Therefore, pick a good product like VASELINE or ZINC OXIDE paste; it will coat the area just as well as any of the other products and it doesn't cost so much. You can also use one of the baby powders to sprinkle on the affected area, after applying the cream. The powder will absorb excess wetness and thus prevent irritation. However, be careful when using these powders—some contain MAGNESIUM STEARATE. If inhaled by the child often enough, this chemical could cause a form of pneumonia. And be sure to wipe away the creams and powder from the previous application before applying more. Sometimes bacteria build up under the coating, and if it's not cleaned away each time, a BACTERIAL INFECTION could develop.

As the old saying goes, an ounce of prevention is worth a pound of cure. There are steps you can take in preventing DIAPER RASH. Try to change your child's diaper as often as possible. Leaving a wet diaper on for several hours increases the chance of diaper rash. Diapers should be made of soft material and fastened loosely to prevent chafing. Plastic pants should be worn as seldom as possible, because they prevent moisture from evaporating. Their use at night particularly should be discouraged, because infants often urinate soon after they are put to bed for the night. Make sure the diapered area is completely dry before putting on a clean diaper. Exposing the diaper area to warm, dry air for a few minutes between changes will help to keep the skin dry. (This information also applies to adults and children suffering from prickly heat. Wash the area thoroughly and use some sort of talcum powder to keep the area dry.) And don't worry: Before you know it your child will be toilet-trained and diaper rash will be a thing of the past!

SHAVING RASH

SHAVING RASH is a problem that, obviously, affects more men than women. Often a man develops irritation along the neckline after he shaves. This manifests itself in REDNESS and ITCHING. Shaving rash sometimes happens when one tries to get an extra-close shave. There are some things you can do to prevent it.

First of all, it is always best to shave after you get out of the shower. If you don't shower, be sure to wash your face thoroughly; or soak a washcloth in hot water, ring it out, then place it on the face and hold it there for a couple of minutes. The heat and water actually help soften the beard, making it easier to shave. Sometimes it helps to spread a thin layer of moisturizing cream on the face and neck before applying your shaving cream over it.

Always try to shave in the direction of the beard. When you shave against the grain of the beard, you are more likely to develop a shaving rash and the irritation that goes along with it.

After you're done, wash away the excess lather. It might also help to cleanse your face with an alcoholic astringent such as WITCH HAZEL. It will tighten up the pores and improve your skin tone. You are also wiping away any soapy residue of shaving, which can cause irritation. After drying the face, apply a non-greasy moisturizer to the skin.

After-shave lotions are nice, but some people get carried away with them. A lot of them have alcohol bases that can irritate the skin. If you occasionally break out in a rash after using them, either stop using them altogether or just dab a little on the pulse points. These steps may take a little longer, but they will help cut down on the irritation caused by shaving.

16

EAR PRODUCTS

Ear disorders are very common, and in most cases cause a great deal of discomfort. However, before buying ear drops, you should check with your pharmacist. The symptoms you have will play an important role in choosing the right product. For example, do you have a cold or flu? How long have the symptoms been present? Have you been swimming within the past several days? Do you have a fever? Many disorders of the ear are minor and fairly easily resolved. But some untreated ear problems can result in hearing loss.

Actually there are three different ways to treat ear problems without prescription drugs. The most common ear problems are caused by a build-up of earwax, which in turn causes pressure and pain in the ear. People sometimes stick different objects into the ear to try to break up the earwax and to clean the ear. They use things such as cotton swabs, hairpins, matchsticks, pencils, and fingers, among others. When using objects like these you can scratch the eardrum, forming an opening for germs and infection.

If your pain is caused by hardening of earwax, then you will want to use a product to soften it. One ingredient for that purpose is CARBAMIDE PEROXIDE, which is found in products such as COLUMBIA EAR DROPS, DEBROX DROPS, and EAR DROPS BY MURINE. These products effervesce when placed in the ear, breaking up earwax and debris in the ear. They also release oxygen, which helps heal infected tissue. When you use these drops, tilt your head so that the affected ear faces up. Hold this pose for at least fifteen minutes, so that the drops have time to work. The next step is to remove the loosened earwax. Take a soft rubber syringe (usually this comes with the ear drops) and fill it with lukewarm water. Then, with the affected ear tilted down and over the sink, gently flush the ear with water. This process may be repeated a second time, if necessary. It should not be used on children under twelve years of age.

Another substance that has been used for years to soften earwax is OLIVE OIL, also called SWEET OIL. The oil is first warmed by holding a container of it in a cup of hot tap water; it is then dropped into the ear. The heated oil melts some of the wax or at least softens it, allowing easy removal by flushing out the ear with lukewarm water. Sweet oil is also very useful in relieving ITCHING and BURNING in the ear.

Some ear pain is not caused by a build-up of earwax. It is due to INFLAMMATION of the external ear canal as a result of BACTERIAL INFECTION, which can be treated with another household product—vinegar.

To a solution of one ounce water and one ounce glycerin or alcohol, add two to three drops of white vinegar. Using a dropper, place three to four drops into the affected ear, then plug it with a piece of cotton. Because of its acidity, the vinegar creates an environment in the ear unfriendly to bacteria.

Some ear drops contain BENZOCAINE, which is a topical anesthetic. But benzocaine is too slowly absorbed into the skin and for this reason does not give complete relief from pain, though it is long-acting. According to *Consumer Guide* it is so effective that consumers often avoid seeing their doctor for recurring earache, so benzocaine is no longer included in some ear products. People using products with anesthetics in them should be careful, because they can prevent one from knowing if an ear problem is getting worse.

Another cause of ear discomfort is seasonal; it occurs in the summer, when swimming is popular. SWIMMER'S EAR is the result of water being trapped in the ear, causing a severe earache. Products such as SWIM EAR and EAR-DRY contain BORIC ACID in ALCOHOL. The boric acid works to kill bacteria, while the alcohol mixes with the water trapped in the ear and helps it evaporate.

These products can be used right after swimming each time to prevent swimmer's ear. However, try not to use them too often, because they can dry the ear to the point of causing other problems. Instead, try ear plugs when you go swimming. They last a lot longer than ear drops and do not cause additional problems.

If you do decide to use ear plugs to prevent EARACHES, you will notice that there are two different kinds at the drugstore. One type is RUBBER and is used by people when they go swimming to keep water out of the ear. These can also be used in the shower. The other type of ear plug is made of WAX. It is not used to keep water out of the ear, but to eliminate noise. Work them in the palm of your hand to soften them, then stick them into your ear. They do an excellent job of blocking out noise, which can be useful in helping you sleep if noises keep you awake. They are also helpful if you have a noisy job that causes headaches. So make sure you pick the right ear plug for the job.

In summary, read the labels carefully when buying ear drops, since the ingredients in the drops can make the difference between relieving your earache and wasting your money. Most over-the-counter ear products have been shown to be safe and effective and the choice of a specific product should be based on the symptoms you have. (Here is where your pharmacist can play a major role in helping you select the right products.) If you don't get relief from these products in one to two days, however, or if you develop a fever, check with your doctor. *And remember: never stick anything into your ear smaller than the size of the opening itself!*

17

EYE DROPS

They say that the eyes are the windows to the soul. Well, sometimes those windows can become INFLAMED and IRRITATED. There are a limited number of over-the-counter eye drops which are intended to "get the red out." These are basically safe and are effective in relieving minor eye symptoms such as BURNING, STINGING, ITCHING, TEARING, TIREDNESS, or EYE STRAIN.

These problems are usually relatively painless and any one of the over-the-counter eye drops will help. But if you notice severe pain or blurred vision, don't fool around with eye drops. Check with your doctor, especially if you've had these symptoms for 48 hours or more. The most common symptoms people experience are REDNESS and IRRITATION. These may be caused by a variety of conditions from EYE STRAIN to ALLERGIES.

Redness in the eye is caused by enlarged blood vessels. Most of the eye drops available contain a decongestant such as **PHENYLEPHRINE, NAPHAZOLINE,** and **TETRAHYDROZO-LINE.** These ingredients constrict or tighten up the blood vessels, which in turn clears up the eye. Since most products do contain one of these ingredients, buy the cheapest one. In general, over-the-counter eye drops must be sterile while manufactured. They also have preservatives in them to keep them sterile. It is a good habit, before using an eye drop, to shake the bottle and hold it up to a light to make sure that the solution is perfectly clear and that no particles, such as filaments and fibers, are floating in it. All eye drops have expiration dates on the package, so be sure that the eye drops are not too old. A good, safe rule of thumb is not to use a bottle of eye drops after it has been opened for three months or more. Eye washes, accompanied by a small eye cup, are also available. Fill the eye cup with the eye wash solution, and hold it tightly over the eye. Open your eye and roll it around and from side to side. Eye washes are refreshing to the eye, and they are really useful if you have a foreign particle in the eye. But they are less convenient than the drops.

Sometimes a condition known as PINK EYE may develop, in which the inner lining of the eye becomes inflamed. You can usually clear it up with any one of the over-the-counter eye drops, but sometimes it becomes contagious. When you have a cold or a sinus infection you may rub your nose and then rub your eye. Actually what you are doing is spreading bacteria from the nose to the eye, resulting in classic pink eye. If you notice a GREENISH DISCHARGE in the corner of the eye, check with your doctor immediately: you may have a contagious infection and will probably need an antibiotic eye drop to clear it up.

Wearing eye make-up may make the eyes look great, but removing it can cause irritation, depending on what you use. Some women use soap and water, but soap will burn the eye if it gets in it. If you wear eye make-up, you might want to check the cosmetic area of the drugstore. They have jars of pads for removing eye make-up. These pads are soaked in MINERAL OIL, which is not as irritating to the eye as other substances. It works just as well to use a cotton cleansing pad dipped in plain MINERAL OIL—it is also a lot cheaper.

There are some over-the-counter eye drops purported to kill bacteria. They contain BORIC ACID. However, I don't advise using them—boric acid is very weak at killing bacteria, and it sometimes causes problems, especially in children. Sometimes kids can get into the contents of the bottle of eye drops. Every year there are a number of accidental poisonings in children who drink products like this. Also, since boric acid is a weak antiseptic, if an infection is present it may need a stronger antibiotic. If you keep using the boric acid solution and your infection is getting worse it could permanently damage the eye.

Remember, when using eye drops containing decongestants, to be careful; just as decongestants in nose sprays can cause a REBOUND REACTION, so can those in eye drops. Thus decongestant eye drops constrict the blood vessels, getting rid of redness. But prolonged use may cause the blood vessels to enlarge again in a shorter and shorter period of time. Also, remember that these eye drops are mainly used for cosmetic purposes, to clear the eyes. Prolonged use may actually mask the symptoms of a serious eye problem.

If you suffer from GLAUCOMA or any other chronic eye disease, do not use any product without checking with your pharmacist or doctor first. If you have pain in the eye, you can get temporary relief by taking an oral pain-relieving product, but you should check with your doctor as soon as possible.

18

FEMININE HYGIENE

American society today is probably unsurpassed in its concern for cleanliness, personal hygiene, and elimination of body odor. Vaginal douches are not new, but feminine deodorant sprays are. They were introduced in the 1960s and since that time you can hardly pick up a magazine without seeing advertisements for them. According to the advertisements, you are not clean and refreshed unless you use one of these products. However, most gynecologists believe that the healthy vagina cleanses itself. Although some doctors seem to feel that douching, when done properly, promotes healthy vaginal tissues, the value of feminine deodorant sprays is very controversial. It has been found that the ingredients in douches and deodorants change the natural bacterial environment of the vagina, as do antibiotics. Their effectiveness, whether you use the spray or the powder, is questionable. Nevertheless, doctors are finding more and more women who have used these products and who subsequently develop IRRITATION of the vagina. The deodorant sprays have also been known to cause ALLERGIC REACTIONS in men after intercourse, resulting in IRRITATION, ITCHING, and PULLING of the skin on the penis.

DOUCHES

These are available in liquids, liquid concentrates (which are diluted with water before use), and powders (to be dissolved in water). No matter what product you use, be sure to follow the instructions on the package because of the possibility of local irritation.

Some douches like MASSENGILL DOUCHE POWDER and BO-CAR-AL contain astringents such as AMMONIUM and POTASSIUM ALUMS and are used to reduce local SWELLING and INFLAMMATION. Other douche products contain BORIC ACID or an iodine product such as BETADINE and are used to stop bacterial infections. If you notice signs of IRRITATION and ITCHING, try a douche with an ingredient to kill bacteria. If the infection is too far advanced, these products will not help much because of their low concentrations. It would be best to check with your doctor.

If you do use douche products, there are a few things to keep in mind.

- Excessive pressure should never be used in giving douches. The force of gravity is sufficient to create a flow of the douche into the vagina if a bag, tube, and nozzle are used.
- Water used to dilute the powder or liquid concentrate should be lukewarm and not hot.
- Douching equipment should be cleaned thoroughly before and after use.
- Douches should not be used during pregnancy.
- A douche should not be used after using a contraceptive foam or suppository, because it will wash away some of the spermicide that serves as a protective barrier against impregnation.

FEMININE DEODORANT SPRAYS

These are aerosol products intended to be used on the external genital area to reduce or mask objectionable odor.

They are available in mist or powder form. If these products are held too close to the skin while spraying, they can cause IRRITATION and SWELLING of tissues. If you decide to use one of these products, be sure to hold it six to eight inches away from your body. And if you notice a STINGING or BURNING sensation when you use it, or if ITCHING develops, stop using it before your problem becomes a lot worse.

MENSTRUAL PAIN RELIEVERS

MENSTRUATION is a fact of life for women during their child-bearing years. At this point in a woman's cycle she may experience PAIN, FLUID ACCUMULATION, BACKACHES, BREAST TENDERNESS, IRRITABILITY, ABDOMINAL CRAMPING, ANXIETY, and DEPRESSION. It is therefore not surprising that many women are a little "on edge" during this period. The severity of the symptoms varies considerably from individual to individual. There are a number of over-the-counter products made specifically to treat these symptoms. Some products are simple pain-relievers and contain ASPIRIN, PHENACITIN, ACETAMINOPHEN, or SALICYLAMIDE. However, aspirin is probably the best choice of ingredients because it relieves INFLAMMATION. You may take one or two tablets of aspirin every four to six hours. However, if you suffer from CHRONIC STOMACH PROBLEMS, or if your stomach is acting up because of menstruation, you might want to use one of the acetaminophen products like TYLENOL or DATRIL. These probably won't work quite as well as aspirin, but they won't upset the stomach as much. Some premenstrual aids, such as MIDOL, contain an ANTIHISTAMINE, such as METHAPYRILENE or PHENINDAMINE, along with a pain reliever. The antihistamine causes drowsiness, so if your symptoms are NERVOUSNESS and TENSION, these products might help to some degree.

Some women suffer swelling in the hands and feet during their periods. They may feel bloated. A product with a mild DIURETIC may help relieve this problem to some degree. Such products contain PAMABROM, CAFFEINE, and AMMO-

NIUM CHLORIDE. However, these only help get rid of water in the body to a small degree, not as effectively as prescription diuretics would. Still, they may give you enough relief to get you through your period with the least amount of discomfort. It also helps to stay away from salt and salt-rich foods, such as pickles and snack chips, during your period.

If you are troubled routinely you might want to talk to your doctor about taking a prescription diuretic. There are also some new pain-relieving prescriptions on the market today that work well at relieving menstrual pain; we will have a lot more to say about those products in our next book on prescription drugs. One of the most effective treatments of backaches and cramping is a combination of dolomite (a naturally occurring calcium compound) and cod liver oil capsules (these contain vitamin A, which is necessary for the body to metabolize calcium). The backaches and cramps result from a decrease in usable calcium; dolomite helps restore the balance. Dolomite is available in health food stores and some drugstores and should be taken a few days before the onset of the period, when the first symptoms appear, through the days of heaviest flow.

Also, herb teas (some specially formulated for the purpose) act as an effective diuretic, without harming the kidneys, as prescription and nonprescription diuretics do. Mild exercise is helpful in relieving pelvic congestion.

Many misconceptions still exist regarding limitations in one's daily activities during menstruation. One of the most common misconceptions is that women should not bathe or wash themselves during this time. Good hygiene that includes routine showering or bathing is one of the most effective ways of reducing menstrual odors. Various feminine products including towelettes, sprays, and douches are marketed to assist the menstruating female in her personal hygiene. (See earlier discussion of the limitations of these products.) Menstrual discomfort is a part of the lives of many American women; while it is inconvenient, the discomfort is rarely so severe as to prevent a woman from carrying out her daily activities. Also many over-the-counter products work to relieve various symptoms to some degree.

SANITARY NAPKINS AND TAMPONS

Years ago there were only two brands of sanitary napkins, KOTEX and MODESS. I remember these products well, because one of my first jobs in the drugstore was to wrap the boxes in plain paper. Back then, women were embarrassed to be seen buying these products. For a long time, there was only one brand of tampon, TAMPAX, which received the same treatment. Nowadays we have all sorts of products, ranging from sanitary napkins and tampons to panty shields and liners, and they are displayed right out in the open.

Recently there has been much media coverage of a serious illness called TOXIC SHOCK SYNDROME, which was associated with the use of tampons. It caused many deaths. Even though we have only recently heard of this problem, I am sure that it has been around since the first tampon was developed.

Toxic Shock Syndrome is believed to be caused by bacteria that gets into the bloodstream, causing a bacterial infection. This bacterial infection was found among women who used tampons, particularly a brand called RELY, which has since been removed from the market by the manufacturer. However, there are still many other brands of tampons on the market and a lot of women use them because of their comfort and convenience. You at least should be aware that if you develop symptoms such as FEVER, CHILLS, MUSCLE ACHES, and NAUSEA while wearing them, you should contact your doctor immediately. If the symptoms are a sign of a bacterial infection due to wearing tampons, the longer you wait the more severe the infection can become, causing a serious hazard to your health. Do not pass these symptoms off as the flu if you currently are wearing tampons.

19

FEVER BLISTERS

This is one condition that makes you want to go around with your hand over your mouth, because you don't want anyone to see you have a nasty ol' fever blister. Meanwhile everyone is probably thinking that you have bad breath. Many people think that fever blisters are caused by the sun, or a cold, or other conditions. Actually they are caused by a virus, which may be triggered by some of the conditions just mentioned. When we are out in the sun, the sun actually dries out the lips, and this dryness of the lips is a good environment for the virus to grow in. Before you know it you've got one or more fever blisters. If you notice that they develop after being out in the sun, coat your lips with any sort of cream to keep them moist.

Some people develop fever blisters when they have a cold. Nasal congestion often causes them to breathe through their mouths, which in turn dries out the lips. Also, the fever that sometimes accompanies a cold may cause the lips to dry out. Again, try coating the lips with a little VASELINE during the course of your illness.

Once you develop a fever blister, as with any virus, you simply have to let it run its course, which is usually about seven to ten days. But there are some products on the market that might be useful in cutting down that time period.

SPIRITS OF CAMPHOR and CAMPHO-PHENIQUE are useful in treating fever blisters and cold sores because they help dry them out. But they also may cause the sores to form a hard scab on the lip, which may then crack open the scab when the mouth is opened, causing pain and discomfort.

Other products are intended to coat the fever blister and keep it soft, so that it is not so painful. Products like BLISTEX and BLISTER KLEAR are in cream form. There are also lip balms, such as CHAPSTICK, BLISTIK, and VASELINE INTENSIVE CARE lip balm, which work the same way. Since they are in a tube similar to lipstick they are probably a little more convenient to use. When you apply any of these products, be sure to cover the cold sore or fever blister completely, especially during the first two or three days when it is contagious and could spread.

Also available without a prescription is an oral tablet called LYSINE 500 mg., of which you take three tablets a day for four to five days. People taking it say that it cuts down on the amount of time they have the fever blister. LYSINE tablets are nothing more than an AMINO ACID, or protein; therefore it is safe. If you suffer from fever blisters quite often, you might want to check into this product.

Another new product is HERPECIN-L, which should be used at the point at which you feel ITCHING and BURNING of the lips. It contains ingredients that help kill the virus at its earliest stages. This product is in the form of a lipstick.

CANKER SORES

These differ from fever blisters in that they develop on the inside of the mouth. They usually appear in groups and most often are limited to the inside of the cheek and lips, though occasionally they form on the tongue and roof of the mouth. The sore is usually round or oval in shape and white in color. Canker sores are not contagious. The cause of canker sores is not known, but it has been shown that people tend to develop them during times of physical and emotional stress. Also certain foods seem to trigger canker sores. Women tend to develop them more than men. One of two kinds of treatment is possible: You can use one of the products for toothache or sore gums that contain a numbing ingredient, such as ORAJEL, NUMZIDENT, or BENZODENT, and this would help stop the pain associated with a canker sore. You could also use one of the PEROXIDE GELS such as GLY-OXIDE or PROXIGEL. They release oxygen at the site of the sore, which in turn helps to heal it. Try to stay away from acidic foods while you have one, because they will irritate the sore.

HERPES SIMPLEX

Infections caused by HERPES SIMPLEX viruses are now epidemic; more than five million people in the United States alone suffer with GENITAL HERPES and many more suffer with LABIAL HERPES, which affects lips, mouth, and face. Both forms can be annoyingly recurrent and disruptive, and both are highly contagious when active sores are present.

Herpes is caused by a virus. The virus enters your body when you come into direct contact with someone who is infected. Once the virus is established in your body and an active infection develops, you are capable of passing the virus to another person.

Typically, a herpes infection appears two to twenty days after exposure. It takes the form of sores on or around the lips, mouth, face, or on or around the sex organs. These sores may ITCH, BURN, or be quite PAINFUL. They may be accompanied by SWOLLEN GLANDS, general MUSCLE ACHES, and sometimes a FEVER. The sores may last for two to three weeks and then heal completely. This marks the end of the active phase of herpes. The virus, however, is still present in your body and enters a dormant phase. Some persons never experience a recurrence following the initial infection, some only infrequently, others quite regularly.

Herpes can be treated and cared for, but at present, not cured. Treatment and care are directed toward relieving the pain, itching, and burning of active sores and preventing their becoming further infected. Bathing with soap and water or other drying agents, such as EPSOM SALTS or BURROWS SOLUTION, is helpful in preventing the sores from becoming infected and may speed the drying up of the sores. Herpes is highly contagious when the sores are present, and one should not allow them to come into contact with another person. Not only can the virus be transmitted to another person, but by touching a sore and then touching some other part of your body you can move the virus to a new location. This is especially true during the initial episode of the disease. Fingers and eyes are particularly vulnerable, so exercise great caution and wash after deliberately or accidentally touching the sores.

If you develop any sort of sore after coming into contact with another person, it would be a good idea to check with your doctor both to determine what it is and to cope with it.

20
FIRST AID

Accidents have a way of happening when you least expect them. The incidence of minor cuts and scrapes increases when the kids are home, playing, running, or riding their bikes, and may send you running to the Corner Drugstore to buy a week's supply of Band-Aids. First aid is everybody's responsibility. Being ready to give emergency care can make the critical difference in saving a life, relieving pain, or preventing further injury or infection. Mothers, since they are most often home with the kids, soon become household paramedics whether they want to or not.

Here are some first-aid tips on some of the most common minor injuries:

- For first- or second-degree burns, the first step is to run cold water over the area. Cold water is preferable to ice, but if ice is the only thing available, use it. Keep the burned area submerged as long as you feel pain. The sooner you get the area into cool water, the sooner you'll get relief; it could also mean the difference between redness of the skin and a blister.

- To stop a nose bleed, have the victim sit quietly with his or her head forward and nostrils pressed together.
- To give first aid for a bruise, apply ice or cold cloths as soon as the injury happens.
- To give first aid for a bruise a few hours after the injury, apply warm, wet cloths, or any other type of heat treatment.
- A frostbitten area should be soaked first in water that is lukewarm, not hot, with the temperature very gradually increased.
- If you are called upon to give first aid for bleeding, first apply direct pressure to the cut.
- To remove a speck of dirt from someone's eye, wash it with clean water.
- For a minor cut the first thing to do, if you possibly can, is to wash it with soap and water. Remember, if the injury is severe, or if there is any doubt in your mind about how severe it is, *call the doctor or get to an emergency room.*

When people come into the drugstore to pick up Band-Aids, gauze, and tape to wrap wounds, they often want to know what is good to put on the cut as a dressing. Nowadays we have ANTIBIOTIC CREAMS, HYDROCORTISONE CREAMS, FIRST-AID CREAMS, and of course the old stand-bys TINCTURE OF MERTHIOLATE and TINCTURE OF IODINE. I remember as a kid that these products always brought their share of screams and yells when they were applied to a cut. But here's the funny thing: When you go to the drugstore to buy iodine or merthiolate, you will see that they are available in both solution and tincture forms. Tincture means that alcohol is the base and it is alcohol that causes the burning. Solution means the ingredient is dissolved in water. Mom, you'll be a real hit with the kids if you use a solution, because it doesn't burn. Boy! I wish my parents knew that when I was a kid.

Most doctors will tell you that washing with soap and

water is adequate to treat a minor cut. However, if you decide to apply a dressing, the antibiotic creams will prevent INFECTION. Be sure to apply these products on and around the cut to prevent germs from getting to it. Three of the most commonly used creams are NEOSPORIN, NEO-POLYCIN, and MYCITRACIN. However, there are other products that work just as well. Since these products contain antibiotics to stop infection, the creams and ointments will have an expiration date on the package. Make sure the product you're buying is not outdated, and be sure to replace your old tube with a new supply.

Other creams that are available are mainly intended to soothe and coat the affected area, including JOHNSON AND JOHNSON first aid cream. By the way, Johnson and Johnson now offers step-by-step directions for treating minor injuries on the backs of some of their products. In addition they provide a toll-free number on the boxes of certain bandages in case you have a question about their use.

Another group of products that is very effective for treating MINOR CUTS and SCRATCHES, INSECT BITES, and RASHES are the HYDROCORTISONE creams such as CORTAID or CLEARAID. Cortisone, which is naturally produced in the body, plays an important role in wound healing.

You also can buy first-aid kits in the drugstore, which have everything you'll need. Unfortunately they often contain things you'll never use as well. You can make your own first-aid kit to keep at home and carry in your car on trips. Find a plastic container with a lid, preferably one that is airtight. The kit should include an assortment of adhesive pads, six yards of sterile gauze bandage (the two-inch width is the most generally useful), adhesive tape, individual towelettes (either the alcohol or antiseptic type), antibiotic ointment, antihistamine tablets, and one of the hydrocortisone creams. Also, it is a good idea to include aspirin, tweezers, and a needle for removing splinters, a single-edge razor blade, scissors, a laxative, and a first-aid booklet. Always carry some loose change in case you need to make an emergency phone call while on a trip. These items will cover

most minor injuries. It is also important to know what each
of the items in your kit is used for, and when to use them.
If you are going to be in an area where snakes are prevalent,
then your kit should include a snake-bite kit. Or if you are
highly allergic to bee or wasp stings an ANA KIT should be
included. If you are a diabetic you may want to keep some
sugar handy. It probably is a good idea to keep an extra bottle of insulin around for emergency purposes such as breaking your other bottle of insulin. Just make sure that it is
stored properly so it doesn't go bad or outdate. If you keep
an extra bottle of insulin in case of an accident with your
regular supply, use your spare bottle next and then replace
the spare bottle with a newly purchased bottle. That way
you are keeping your insulin as fresh as possible. Start with
the basic items and add to the kit according to your own
needs or the area you are going to.

ATHLETIC SUPPLIES

Last year, over 20 million sports-related injuries were
reported in the United States. The most frequently inju-
rious sport was bicycling, followed by baseball, football, and
basketball. However, roller skating, a recent sports fad, is
rapidly gaining on the list of injury-prone sports.

Since many schools have increased their emphasis on
physical education, Mom and Dad are kept busy patching
up those minor injuries the kids come home with. Many
pharmacies have set up areas featuring various types of athletic supplies, including athletic supporters and braces for
the knee, elbow, foot, or ankle. As a matter of fact, there is
even a special kind of brace to prevent tennis elbow.

Since most sports injuries are strains, sprains, or bruises,
here is a good rule of thumb for treating those injuries,
based on the word ICE.

I   stands for ice. Apply ice to the injured area as
        soon as possible after the injury happens.

C   is for compression. After soaking the injured
     area in ice, wrap it with an elastic bandage.
E   is to remind you to keep the injured area ele-
     vated as much as possible.

Nowadays there are a wide variety of ice bags to choose
from. The most familiar and fittingly named one is the kind
that you add ice cubes to. Another type has a gel in it and
can be used as either a hot or a cold pack, by placing the
package in the freezer or in warm water. The chemical ice
pack is a package that has two separate chemicals in it.
When you use it, simply puncture the inner package and
the two chemicals mix together, producing a cold pack.

You may also take a pain reliever such as ASPIRIN, which
will help relieve the INFLAMMATION causing the pain. It also
may help in stopping cartilage damage.

In order to cut down on the number of injuries, it is best
to wear the proper type of equipment, such as braces, supporters, even goggles. Also, a good stretching program, both
before and after exercise, is important to prevent sports
injuries.

21

FOOT CARE PRODUCTS

As the old saying goes, when your feet hurt you feel bad all over. Although foot conditions generally are not life-threatening (except perhaps in diabetics), foot problems cause their share of pain and discomfort. Some common conditions that people suffer from are CORNS, CALLUSES, BUNIONS, and WARTS.

CORNS AND CALLUSES

A corn is a raised, yellowish-gray area on the foot that has a central core. Corns are either hard or soft. Hard corns occur on the surfaces of the toes and appear very shiny. Soft corns are a thickening of the skin, usually found on the webs between the fourth and fifth toes.

A callus differs from a corn in that it has no central core and is much thicker. Callouses form on weight-bearing areas (such as the palms of the hands and the sides and soles of the feet).

The successful treatment of corns and calluses really depends on eliminating the causes, such as pressure and friction. One way of doing that is to buy well-fitted, non-binding footwear that distributes body weight evenly.

Corns can also be treated by using medicated corn pads. The pads usually are available along with a medicated disc that is put directly on the corn itself. The disc contains SALICYLIC ACID, which is responsible for removing dead tissue. While the medicated disc works on the removal of the corn, the pad surrounds the corn, keeping the pressure off. Liquid corn removers also have salicylic acid as the main ingredient. Simply apply a few drops to the corn itself. Avoid putting these products on healthy tissue nearby; it may cause IRRITATION. Some corn and callus removers have an ingredient called ZINC CHLORIDE, which is even more irritating and caustic than salicylic acid. Be careful when using it and do not use it for long periods of time.

Calluses can be handled in one of two ways: a pressure-relieving pad will stop the build-up of dead tissue, and products containing salicylic acid or zinc chloride will remove some of the layers of tissue, which in turn will reduce pressure. When a person has a callus, the thickened skin can actually crack or split open, causing pain. One way to handle that is by reducing the callus with a file. Callus files may be found in the foot care section of the drugstore. They do the same job as the corn and callus removers, without chemicals. It is best to do your filing when the foot is dry. Afterwards apply a lotion (any type of moisturizing cream or lotion will do) to the area to reduce the irritation from filing.

An old home remedy for corns and calluses is CASTOR OIL. As a matter of fact it is still used in some of the products available today. Actually it does nothing to remove corns and calluses; it simply keeps the tissue soft and pliable. The oil is usually applied at bedtime; the foot is then covered with a sock to prevent the oil from staining the bed linens and to help the castor oil penetrate deeper. However, since castor oil does not remove the excess layers of skin that cause the problem, it is simply a treatment to give relief. When you see the price of castor oil, however, I think you'll agree that you are better off with a different, and more effective, product.

BUNIONS

This is a swelling that occurs along the side of the big toe. They are usually caused by pressure from a tightly fitting shoe, but they may also be caused by pressure resulting from the way a person sits, stands, or walks. Treatment of BUNIONS often depends on the degree of discomfort you have. Bunions can become PAINFUL, SWOLLEN, and TENDER. Most over-the-counter products do not alter this condition at all. The only thing you can use is a bunion pad, which may give you relief. If it does not, surgery may be required. Remember, if you do use a bunion pad, wear a slightly larger-sized shoe or slipper to avoid pressure.

WARTS

Warts, regardless of what you have heard, are not caused by frogs. They are actually caused by viruses. Warts are common in children and young adults and usually appear on exposed areas of the fingers, hands, face, and soles of the feet. Warts that appear on the soles of the feet are called PLANTARS WARTS. Sometimes they go unnoticed, but if they get large and begin causing a great deal of discomfort, check with your doctor. Since warts are caused by viruses they may, over a period of time, go away by themselves. Among the products that are available to treat warts are COMPOUND W, VERGO ointment, or MOSCO. COMPOUND W and MOSCO contain SALICYLIC ACID, a compound you are probably familiar with by now, and they remove tissue. VERGO ointment contains CALCIUM PANTOTHENATE, which aids in removal of the wart as well as relief of ITCHING. This product is generally recommended for children. Treatment of warts is extremely difficult. Warts may reappear several months after they supposedly have been cured no matter what procedure you use for removal.

When using any sort of over-the-counter product to remove corns, calluses, or warts, try to soak the affected area throughout the treatment period for at least five minutes a day in very warm (not hot) water to remove dead tissue. If you are using one of the liquid removers, an application of VASELINE to the healthy skin surrounding the area, before applying the medicine, will protect the healthy skin.

DIABETES

Diabetics should be cautioned before using any foot product. Since their circulation in the feet and legs is usually not very good, any sort of foot sore may be very difficult to heal and may even cause severe bacterial infections. This very definitely means do not attempt "bathroom surgery" on the feet or toe nails using sharp knives or razor blades. In some cases diabetics have poor eyesight, which increases the chance of a serious mishap.

If you do suffer from DIABETES, or POOR CIRCULATION, at least talk it over with your doctor or pharmacist before you use any product for your feet.

FOOT ODOR

Remember the television commercial in which the guy took off his shoes and the dog fell over? Well, no one is immune to foot odor, unless of course you don't wear any shoes at all. If you have this problem, you will certainly want to use something to get rid of it. Foot odor is caused by the feet sweating inside one's shoes. Bacteria attack the perspiration, and the resulting decomposition of the sweat leads to foot odor. There are products in the foot care section of most drugstores to help you. These are usually available in aerosol cans. Some are nothing more than a fragrance, and these will not do an effective job. Other products, called "foot refreshers," contain CAMPHOR and MENTHOL and are intended to be sprayed on tired feet to give a cooling effect. To combat foot odor, look for the foot spray with the word *antiperspirant*. Such a product works just like your underarm deodorant and is intended to keep the feet from sweating, which in turn prevents odor. You might even try your underarm antiperspirant on your feet if it is the aerosol spray kind.

You will also notice foot powders in the foot care section. They work to lessen foot odor by absorbing perspiration that develops. Alternatively, you might sprinkle a little BAKING SODA in your shoes since it also works very well at eliminating odor.

If you don't want to use a powder in your shoe, you might try one of the insoles that are available, such as ODOR EATERS or DOCTOR SCHOLL'S. They contain CHARCOAL, which absorbs perspiration. Like anything else, they do have to be replaced periodically. As to the question of when to replace them, don't worry: You'll be the first to know.

ATHLETE'S FOOT

Everyone is becoming very exercise-minded nowadays. People are out jogging or playing tennis and racquetball. You come home, kick off your tennis shoes, rub your toes in the carpet, and suddenly you notice some ITCHING or REDNESS between the toes. My friend, you may not have the talent of an athlete, but you do have his feet: that is, ATHLETE'S FOOT. Athlete's foot may occur at any age, but it is more common in adults. Athlete's foot is a FUNGUS INFECTION most often acquired by walking barefoot on infected floors in bathrooms, locker rooms, and camps. This fungus infection can spread to other members of the family via the bathroom floor, floor mats, or rugs. The main complaint of people suffering from athlete's foot is severe ITCHING, although sometimes cracks develop between the toes that cause painful BURNING and STINGING. There are many different products to treat athlete's foot, and they are available in many forms as well, including creams, ointments, liquids, and powders. They contain one or more of the following ingredients:

UNDECYLENIC ACID is an active ingredient in DESENEX, which is available in liquid, ointment, and powder and is effective in mild cases of athlete's foot. It is applied directly to the affected area. However, if the skin is broken the liquid form will burn because it is in an alcoholic base. Always make sure that these products do not come into contact with the eyes. They are usually applied twice a day and you should notice improvement in two to four weeks. If there is no improvement, check with your doctor or pharmacist.

TOLNAFTATE is sold under the trade names of TINACTIN or AFTATE. Tolnaftate is one of the most effective anti-fungal agents that can be applied to the skin. It is available in aerosol, liquid, cream, and powder form and is applied twice a day. Usually you can see results in two to four weeks, but some cases may take four to six weeks, especially when LESIONS are present between the toes.

There are other products available to treat athlete's foot, but they don't work quite as well to effectively kill the fungus that causes the problem. Since many of these products are available in powder form, it might be a good idea to use one of them after you apply a liquid or cream to provide continuous release of medicine and to absorb moisture from the feet. However, be careful if you are inclined to use powder as a primary treatment, especially if you have broken skin. Some powders contain boric acid, which should not be absorbed into the skin.

JOCK ITCH

JOCK ITCH is also caused by a fungus growth, usually in

the groin area and on the inner folds of the legs, and resulting in severe ITCHING. Sometimes the skin breaks open and on hot, sweaty days there can be additional irritation. The best thing to do is to wash the area thoroughly and as often as possible. After washing, apply one of the anti-fungal powders such as TINACTIN or AFTATE. It will kill the fungus and stop it from spreading. The powder also absorbs perspiration to prevent further irritation. Remember, you don't have to be a jock or even play sports to be bothered by this problem. The main thing is to know when you have it and how to effectively treat it.

SUPPORT STOCKINGS

These products are usually found near the foot care products, but people don't know much about them. VARICOSE VEINS are a problem that many people, mostly women, suffer from. The condition is caused by sitting or standing too long in the same position. Blood flowing too slowly through an artery causes it to bulge out. Some people simply complain that their legs feel tired all the time. This could be caused by POOR CIRCULATION. In either case, your doctor may suggest that you wear a support stocking. Don't be put off by this; support stockings are no longer ugly and unfashionable. In fact they are available in styles and colors to complement any wardrobe. There are even support panty hose. Do talk it over with your pharmacist if you plan to buy support stockings. In order to get the right size, you need accurate measurements of the foot and the leg. If you simply select a pair that is the same size you normally wear, you may be getting one that fits the calf muscle too loosely and will do you no good at all. On the other hand, if you have large calf muscles, you may get a pair that fits too tightly, which could cut off the circulation completely. This is especially important if you have a job where you sit or stand for long periods of time.

A new product that has come on the market recently is

an electric foot massager. To operate, fill the unit with water, plug it in, then place your feet in the water. Vibrations on the bottom of the feet help increase circulation in the feet, which results in their feeling refreshed. Provided you are not ticklish, if you have a job where you stand a lot, you might want to try one of these foot massagers. You may find it a very relaxing way to unwind after a hard day, as well as to take care of tired, sore feet.

If you don't want to invest in one of these products, try soaking your feet in a tub of warm water and one or two ounces of EPSOM SALTS. If that helps your feet, fine! But just think how much better they would feel with a massage on top of soaking them. However, it is not a good idea to add anything to the water in these machines, unless the manufacturer of the machine indicates that it is safe to do so. A build-up of chemicals could interfere with the proper working of the machine.

22

GADGETS

We have all heard the expression "It's a hard pill to swallow." Well, some people do have a hard time taking tablet and capsule forms of medicines. In many drugstores, usually near the prescription counter, there are all kinds of gadgets to make taking medicine easier. For liquid medicines, there is a gadget composed of a calibrated tube with a spoon on one end. Simply pour the medicine into the tube up to the teaspoon mark, then place the other spoon end in the child's mouth to deliver the right amount of medicine each time. For people who have trouble swallowing tablets and capsules, there is the Drink-a-Pill, manufactured by the Apex Medical Company. This gadget is a plastic cup with a ledge just inside the lip. Fill the cup with water, then place your pills on the ledge. You then drink the water and let nature take its course. As the water goes down, so do the pills. You won't even notice it.

For people who have difficulty remembering to take their medicine each day, there is a pill box with seven compartments, each one marked with the day of the week. This system helps you keep track of whether you have or have not taken your medicine on a particular day. Also available are the fancy little pill boxes that some people carry their med-

icine in. I don't advise using them because they do not provide an air-tight container, and medicines often lose their
potency much faster when they are exposed to air. Also,
since these containers do not have a prescription label, if
any accident or emergency occurs, it will take doctors
longer to find out what medicines you have been taking
before they begin treatment on you. As a matter of fact,
some people have had problems with the authorities when
they found an unlabeled container of drugs in their posses-
sion. So if you do carry your medicine with you, don't take
any chances. Carry your medicine in its original bottle with
the prescription label intact. It could be life-saving in an
emergency situation or keep you out of an awkward one.

Some pharmacies carry a plastic cigarette called SMOKE
BREAK, to be used by people who want to cut down on cigarette smoking. You just pretend that it's a real cigarette,
keep it in your mouth, or hold it between your fingers. (You
could also do this with any thing that resembles a cigarette,
such as a plastic straw.) Cigarettes are a definite health hazard. There are no safe cigarettes, and those with low tar and
nicotine contents offer only a small amount of protection
against the development of lung cancer.

There are other products available to help you kick the
smoking habit. One of them is a product called BANTRON,
which contains an ingredient called LOBILINE. Another is
NIKOBAN. Loboline resembles nicotine chemically. It
seems that when we smoke cigarettes, nicotine gets into the
bloodstream. Because it is addictive, as the nicotine level
drops, we develop an urge for a cigarette, or the so-called
"nicotine fit." A BANTRON tablet puts a substance into your
bloodstream resembling nicotine, which reduces the desire
for a cigarette. These products are non-addictive; once you
have stopped smoking cigarettes long enough, you may stop
taking the tablets and, we hope, will stay away from cigarettes forever.

Some people, instead of cutting out cigarettes completely,
have turned to low tar and nicotine cigarettes. This does not
necessarily result in decreased intake of tar and nicotine,

however, because many people simply either smoke more cigarettes or puff harder to get more out of each one. Other people are turning to a different form of tobacco usage. The "urban cowboy" fad, along with the tobacco industry's use of professional athletes to portray a macho image for chewing tobacco, has resulted in some 22 million people using smokeless tobacco in the United States, according to recent figures. Like smoking cigarettes, chewing tobacco can harm one's health. Of course, unlike cigarettes, since the smoke is not inhaled, it does not cause as much damage to the lungs. But chewing tobacco does contain nicotine, which is absorbed into the bloodstream, resulting in the same negative effects, such as the constant craving as well as an increase in heart rate and blood pressure.

Smokeless tobacco can also lead to ORAL DISEASE and CANCER as a result of the regular direct contact of tobacco with the tissues of the mouth. IRRITATION from frequent contact could cause the gums to recede, thereby exposing tooth roots and increasing the sensitivity of the teeth to heat and cold. All of this damage, along with unsightly tooth discoloration and bad breath, are brought on by tobacco use.

Some smokeless tobaccos contain sugar to make them better tasting and could cause cavities. Snuff dipping and tobacco chewing are not safe alternatives to smoking.

BLOOD PRESSURE KITS

Drugstores carry a wide assortment of home blood pressure kits, with a wide variety of prices as well. It is really not a bad idea to use one of these kits, especially if you have high blood pressure and are taking medicine to keep it under control. Some of the expensive kits provide electronic monitoring of your blood pressure. But you will probably be just as well off with one of the cheaper models. These consist of a stethescope and a pressure gauge (either the mercury type or the kind that fits on the cuff). After you buy it, take it to your doctor's office the next time you have an appointment. Have him check your blood pressure with his equipment, then have him check it with your blood pressure kit, just to make sure that your kit is accurate. If it isn't, take it back and get one that works accurately. Some stores and shopping malls have machines to measure your blood pressure. All you do is place your money in the machine, put your arm in the designated place, and read off your blood pressure. These machines have been found to be inaccurate, since they are not serviced often enough. If you are considering buying one of the home blood pressure kits, check with your pharmacist. He will give you all the information you need, as well as help you select the easiest kind for you to use. However, don't think that a home blood pressure kit will take the place of a periodic check-up with your doctor. You also need the experience that goes with it.

MEDICAL ALERT BRACELETS

You never know when an accident may happen. You may end up in an emergency room unconscious and unable to give vital information to the people waiting to treat you. People suffering from a chronic disease such as diabetes must be treated differently from normal people. People who are taking certain prescription drugs may have a fatal reaction if they are given other drugs. If you are allergic to certain drugs, such as PENICILLIN, you would want the people treating you to know that fact. A medical alert bracelet gives doctors vital information about your medical background that will help them determine the fastest and safest treatment for you. Some bracelets show a phone number that can be called any time to obtain your complete medical background. The bracelets and necklaces also carry the medical alert symbol, which is recognized around the world. If you suffer from a chronic disease, are allergic to certain medicines, or take certain prescription drugs, you should wear the medical alert bracelet. It could save your life.

There are many other products in the drugstore. Take tweezers, for example; it really amazes me to see all the different types, each with its own particular purpose. A tweezer is a good thing to have around for removing splinters or to shape a woman's eyebrows. The main difference among them is in the ends of the tweezers. For splinters, pick one with pointed ends. For eyebrows, choose whichever does the best job for you. There is now an automatic tweezer that is powered by batteries. If you decide to try it, be careful not to injure yourself; it may not be as gentle as your own hand.

23

HAIR REMOVERS

Hair has a mind of its own. It often doesn't grow in places, such as men's heads, where we want it to grow. Or it grows in places where we don't want it at all—for example, women's legs or underarms. The growth of hair is genetically determined. However, hair that is quite normal medically may be cosmetically unappealing. The options for removing unwanted hair are varied. There is no one best way to remove problem hair, and there are no drugs to effectively stop excess hair growth on otherwise healthy people. In general, there are two ways to get rid of hair: permanent or temporary. Temporary hair removal can be done in one of several ways:

SHAVING

This can be done with either a blade and razor or an electric shaver. Shaving is the most popular way for both men and women to temporarily remove unwanted hair. But once you start removing hair by shaving, you are faced with the continuous task of avoiding the nubs of early growth.

There is no medical reason why women troubled by

excessive facial hair should not shave, yet few do. Most women turn to other forms of temporary hair removal, such as depilatories.

DEPILATORIES

Depilatories are chemical agents that dissolve the hair so that it breaks off at the skin's surface. Two popular brands are NEET and NAIR, which are available in creams and foams. Unfortunately, products that weaken the hair can also cause IRRITATION, REDNESS, and DRYING of the skin. As a matter of fact if you have "detergent hands," or if you are sensitive to household cleaners with ammonia or strong soaps, you might well be allergic to depilatories. If you do decide to try one of these products, it would probably be a good idea to first test it on a small area of the skin, before applying it to a large or prominent area. If you notice a reaction, do not use the product; it could create a problem worse than unsightly hair. These depilatories are only intended for the legs and arms and are usually too strong for the face. There are some products that are intended strictly for the face. These products are used two to three times a week. In order to cut down on unnecessary problems, follow the recommended limits closely. After use, wash the area thoroughly and apply any type of lubricating lotion or cream.

WAXES

These products are also available to get rid of hair. They are nothing more than WAX that is heated and then left to cool until you can apply it to your skin without burning it. After the warm wax is applied to the skin it is allowed to further cool and set. When the cooled wax is stripped off quickly in the direction of hair growth, the embedded hairs are pulled out. This method is not very popular, because many people find the procedure painful. I believe this process could be used effectively in wartime to make the enemy talk. The advantage of the waxes over depilatories is that they remove hair for longer periods of time.

BLEACHING

These products contain chemicals to bleach the hair white so that it isn't noticeable. Most bleaches contain PEROXIDE to bleach the hair. This method is preferred by people who want to disguise rather than remove unwanted hair on their faces or arms. It is also the only method of dealing with unwanted hair that is generally recommended for children.

ELECTROLYSIS

There is one reasonably safe way of removing hair permanently. It is called *electrolysis* and actually destroys the hair germ cells by electric current. This procedure does have its drawbacks. First of all you must locate and treat each hair root individually, and that can be time-consuming. There is often some discomfort and reddening around the hair follicle, which may last several hours after the treatment. Permanent scarring of the skin sometimes occurs, and this can happen even with an experienced operator. The best way to find a competent electrologist is to ask your doctor or dermatologist whom they recommend. Be wary of any home electrolysis device. Do-it-yourself electrolysis carries a higher risk of SCARRING and INFECTION.

24

HEMORRHOIDAL PRODUCTS

Hemorrhoids are another condition that many people joke about. But hemorrhoids are no laughing matter; it is one of the most annoying and uncomfortable disorders suffered by Americans. However, many of the symptoms can be self-treated. There are a number of over-the-counter products for relief of the BURNING, PAIN, ITCHING, and BLEEDING of hemorrhoids.

Some of the causes of hemorrhoids are CONSTIPATION and DIARRHEA, COUGHING, SNEEZING, VOMITING, PREGNANCY, and PHYSICAL EXERTION. Thus we are all prime candidates for hemorrhoids.

Pregnancy is by far the most common cause of hemorrhoids in young women. Some of the signs and symptoms are ITCHING, BURNING, PAIN, INFLAMMATION, IRRITATION, SWELLING, and a lot of DISCOMFORT. All of these symptoms can be relieved by self-medication. BLEEDING, SEEPAGE, and PROTRUSION are more serious symptoms that should not be self-medicated.

Over-the-counter preparations are available in creams, ointments, suppositories, and towelettes. Some contain a local anesthetic such as **BENZOCAINE** or **PRAMOXINE HYDROCHLORIDE**. These products are effective at relieving pain, burning, itching, and irritation, although the condition itself is not changed. Also remember that local anesthetics produce allergic reactions in some people. Products like AMERICAINE, LANACANE, and PAZO work very well at relieving discomfort. Some products also have an ingredient that constricts or tightens the blood vessels. Three ingredients that work in this way are EPHEDRINE, EPINEPHRINE and PHENYLEPHRINE. The products that contain these ingredients are most effective at relieving itching due to the swelling of the rectal blood vessels.

Other products contain protectants. These cover the affected area and act to prevent IRRITATION and WATER LOSS from the tissues. They also help protect tissue from additional irritation from fecal matter and air. For example, PREPARATION H OINTMENT and SUPPOSITORY have shark liver oil as the protectant. Other ingredients used for protecting the irritated area are LANOLIN, PETROLATUM (VASELINE), COCOA BUTTER, CALAMINE, and MINERAL OIL. All of these protectants are recommended for both internal and external use, with the exception of GLYCERIN,which is recommended for external use only. Of the recommended protectants, petrolatum is probably the most effective.

Some of the hemorrhoidal products contain an astringent such as HAMAMELIS WATER (Witch Hazel). This is found in TUCKS PADS and PREPARATION H CLEANSING PADS. These products are easy to use to cleanse the area, and since they contain an astringent, will help shrink swollen tissues. As a matter of fact, some women use these pads to tighten up wrinkles on the face. Use them mainly to cleanse the area, prior to applying a cream or ointment.

Hemorrhoidal suppositories are also available and have been used for many years. A suppository helps ease straining at the stool by its lubricating effect. However, suppositories work slowly because they must melt in order to release the active ingredient. PREPARATION H SUPPOSITORIES are very popular. The active ingredient is shark liver oil, which mainly works by protecting the irritated tissue. Other products like PAZO and RECTAL MEDICONE SUPPOSITORIES have a deadening ingredient such as BENZOCAINE. They also have astringents to shrink swollen tissue.

No matter what type of product you use to treat your hemorrhoids, there are a few things to keep in mind: It is a good idea to soak yourself in a tub of hot water for about fifteen to thirty minutes before applying your cream or ointment. The hot water will not only help to relieve the itching and irritation, but also to open the pores of the skin so your medicine is absorbed faster. Also watch what you eat; some foods may aggravate your symptoms, especially those delicious spicy dishes. It also helps to take a stool softener like COLACE periodically. This keeps the stool soft so you don't have strain and cause further irritation.

A good rule of thumb is to select a product with as few ingredients as possible. Don't buy a stimulant laxative if you don't need it; it will only cause further irritation. Select the product that is a plain stool softener, or ask your pharmacist.

25

HOME REMEDIES (FOLK MEDICINE)

Almost all the cities across the country have health food stores with homey signs, and advertisements saying "natural" or "organic," which raise the price of things. A lot of people are confused these days over the terms *natural* and *synthetic*. Most health food advocates define *natural* or *organic* as meaning foods grown without chemical treatment, such as pesticides or chemical fertilizers, etc., thereby implying that chemicals are bad for you. On the other side of the controversy, medical experts refer to herbal remedies as nonsense when compared to modern, potent, and effective drugs. The truth is that many prescription drugs on the market today are of natural origin. So perhaps it is time to take a closer look at some of the old-time home remedies.

CRANBERRY JUICE

This juice can help fight URINARY TRACT INFECTIONS. Cranberry juice is very acid and in turn makes the urine acid, which creates an environment unfriendly to bacteria. Cranberry juice taken in small amounts (two four-ounce glasses a day) in combination with drugs is sometimes recommended by a physician to fight urinary infections.

APPLES

Can an apple a day keep the doctor away? It might for sufferers of DIARRHEA. The fruit works best when it is eaten raw with the skin, which contains PECTIN. Pectin is the same ingredient found in KAOPECTATE. However, in some people apples have the reverse effect.

CAMOMILE TEA

Camomile tea can help soothe indigestion by relaxing muscles and therefore preventing spasms. It also relieves gas. Camomile has been shown to fight intestinal inflammation and also helps you go to sleep at night.

ALOE VERA

An eye-catching house plant with thick fleshy leaves, the aloe can soothe minor burns. The thick jellylike fluid in the leaves can prevent discomfort and blistering if applied immediately after the injury occurs. The fluid hastens healing mainly by aiding circulation of blood to the affected area. It is also found in lotions as a moisturizer for the skin, as well as a sun-screening agent.

SUGAR

As much as one hears about the bad effects of sugar, it does help to stop HICCUPS. Attacks of hiccups can be caused by excessive laughter or rapid eating or drinking, which excites the nerves controlling the diaphragm, causing it to contract involuntarily. There are many folk remedies for hiccups, and if you have one that works for you, keep doing it. But eating a teaspoonful of a granular substance like sugar causes irritation when swallowed. This irritation stops the contractions of the diaphragm.

BAKING SODA

This one product has many uses around the house. We all probably use it to keep the refrigerator, the cat litter box, sink drains, and the bathroom smelling fresh and clean.

But BICARBONATE OF SODA also has medicinal uses. If you have acid indigestion, simply dissolve one teaspoonful in a glass of water and drink it down. It works instantly to neutralize excess acid indigestion. A half cup of baking soda in your bath water helps strip away oils from the skin. A baking soda bath also helps relieve minor skin IRRITATIONS from INSECT BITES or STINGS, SUNBURN, WIND BURN, PRICKLY HEAT, and POISON IVY, OAK, and SUMAC. Or you can make a paste out of it by mixing it with a little water for relief from bee and wasp stings.

You can sprinkle it directly into your shoes as a deodorant powder. Or mix equal parts of BAKING SODA and your favorite TALCUM POWDER and dust it under the arms as a deodorant.

Many of the old home remedies were actually made from various herbs and spices. Some of the plants used in these remedies can be grown in your own backyard. Plants are often effective medicines, if not the only answer to good health, so let's take a look at some of these old herbal medicines.

GINGER

Hot ginger tea was thought to stimulate a delayed menstrual period, especially if it was due to a cold. Ginger tea was also used to help relieve severe menstrual cramps.

CINNAMON

Five drops of cinnamon oil in a tablespoon of water, taken several times a day at the very onset of the flu, was supposed to prevent you from coming down with the flu.

HONEY

Honey was used for fatigue. (The sugar in the honey is immediately absorbed by the body, giving it a lift.) Honey was usually added to a glass of water.

LEMON

Diluted lemonade with no sugar was used to cleanse the system of boils and to help treat other skin problems.

SAGE

Rubbing sage leaves across the teeth was believed not only to cleanse the teeth, but also to make the breath smell sweet.

VINEGAR

Apple cider vinegar was commonly used to relieve indigestion and heartburn.

ONIONS

Eating raw onions increases the flow of urine, so it was a common practice to relieve premenstrual bloating.

Whether these remedies work or not is debatable; some people swear by them. It is up to you, though it never hurts to check with your doctor.

26
INFANT CARE

According to recent statistics the 1980s will show an increase in births. And it is already happening—more than three-and-one-half million babies will be born in the United States this year, up approximately 150,000 from 1979. More babies mean more diapers, wipes, formulas, bottles, humidifiers, vaporizers, and so on.

Since more and more women are returning to breast feeding, preparing their own foods, and leaning away from prepared infant foods, new products have been developed for this market. Among them are nursing pads, breast pumps, nipple shields, breast creams, and specialized bottles and nipples.

Breast pumps are available in different styles. One type is used to remove milk to reduce the pain and discomfort due to the build-up of milk in the breast. The other type has a bottle attached to it; as you remove the breast milk, it goes into the bottle to be fed to the infant later. This is helpful if you are going to be out somewhere and nursing would be really inconvenient for you.

Often women who are nursing develop sore nipples. There are special creams available to help relieve the irritation, such as **MASSE NIPPLE CREAM.** Also, when breast feeding, you might want to use a nursing pad that you place inside your bra to absorb any leakage.

INFANT FORMULA

Even with the growing trend toward breast feeding, the proportion of breast-fed infants throughout the population remains constant at about 20 percent. Therefore, infant formulas continue to serve a very large market, and you will find a number of different products to satisfy your infant's appetite and nutritional needs.

In evaluating an infant formula, remember that human milk is the standard to which all formulas are compared. Three basic nutritional principles should be considered: The formula should have enough nutrients, be easily digested, and have a balanced distribution of calories from CARBOHYDRATES, PROTEINS, and FATS. Your infant pediatrician will be able to advise you on a suitable formula. Some of the standard formulas commonly used are ADVANCE, ENFAMIL, ENFAMIL WITH IRON, SIMILAC, SIMILAC WITH IRON, and SMA. Most of them use LACTOSE as a source of carbohydrates, COW'S MILK as a source of protein, and SOY and COCONUT OILS as a source of fat. Some premature infants may develop an intolerance to the lactose, causing CRAMPING and DIARRHEA.

The digestibility of the product is important not only to the infant, but also to the parents, as it helps to eliminate wet shirts and blouses. Most commercial formulas have replaced BUTTER FAT with VEGETABLE OILS. Of these, CORN and SOY are easier to digest than COCONUT OIL, so refer to the list of ingredients on the container. Adequate fat in the diet ensures the absorption of the fat-soluble vitamins. Infants should not be given additional vitamins if an infant formula with iron is used, unless they are being used to correct a deficiency.

Because of the prevalence of MILK ALLERGIES, there is some variations in the ingredients used in infant formulas.

Soy is often used instead of milk for protein; some formulas have a particular form of soy protein that is more palatable than others, such as ISOMIL, PRO-SOBEE, and NURSOY. Occasionally infants develop an allergy to the soy. In that case, there are other infant formulas that use different sources of protein (hydrolized casein) including NUTRAMIGEN, PREGESTIMIL, and MEAT-BASED FORMULA (which uses beef heart as a protein source).

The important thing to keep in mind is that if your infant develops such symptoms as CRAMPING, GAS, and DIARRHEA while feeding on infant formula, check with your doctor. Your infant may not be able to tolerate that particular formula. At that point your doctor may recommend a different formula that does agree with your baby.

FEEDING EQUIPMENT

There is a wide variety of equipment available to aid in feeding the infant. Among them are glass and plastic bottles in both four-ounce and eight-ounce sizes. PLAYTEX offers disposable bottles. There are specialized nipples; nipples for milk, juice, and medicine, and even orthodontic nipples. Some nipples resemble breast nipples. If you are using infant formula to feed your child, aside from bottles and nipples you will need bottle brushes, bottle warmers, electric sterilizers, and nipple brushes. It is very important to keep the equipment used in preparing the infant formula as clean as possible. If bacteria builds up and comes into contact with the baby, it may cause such problems as DIARRHEA.

DIAPERS AND WIPES

Diapers should be made of a soft material and loosely fitted to prevent rubbing. It is important to change diapers frequently to prevent DIAPER RASH. You should not use plastic pants routinely. They trap moisture in the diaper, so that if there is any irritation it doesn't heal properly.

The new disposable diapers are convenient and easy to use. Mothers have hailed them as a godsend. When you remove them, you simply throw them away. No more washing diapers in special detergents and then drying and folding them. Products like KLEENEX HUGGIES, LUVS, and PAMPERS have an absorbent layer of material covered by a thin layer of material designed to keep the wetness away from the child.

Disposable diapers are not the answer to diaper rash, because diaper rash is caused by ammonia, heat, and chemical irritants. These products may help keep an infant drier, but they also contain chemicals that can cause further irritation to the affected area. And since disposable diapers have a plastic outer covering, you may not notice that the child is wet as quickly as you would with a cloth diaper. Whether you are using disposable diapers or regular cloth diapers, the same rule applies: Change the infant as soon and as often as possible.

DIAPER RASH

The best therapy for DIAPER RASH and PRICKLY HEAT is to keep the skin dry. Diaper rash is caused by ammonia, sweat retention, and mechanical and chemical irritants. Breast-fed infants tend to urinate less frequently and have a lower incidence of diaper rash.

Mild forms of diaper rash are best treated by changing diapers frequently and leaving them off during naps. It is also a good idea to apply a protective ointment, cream, or powder to the diapered area every time you change the child. If you do so, be sure to wipe away the excess cream from the time before, because bacteria can build up on the cream or powder.

After you remove the excess cream or powder, cleanse

the area thoroughly before reapplying it, using one of the pre-moistened towelettes such as WASH UP, WET ONES, and JOHNSON'S BABY WASH CLOTHS. If these are not available, use plain soap and water. But be sure the soap is not irritating or drying the skin. Your best bet would be to use a soap especially designed for infants' skin, such as JOHNSON'S BABY SOAP or IVORY.

TEETHING LOTIONS

Babies cry for a variety of reasons. One of those reasons is teething, which can send Mom off in a hurry to buy products such as DR. HAND'S TEETHING LOTION, NUMZIT, and ORAJEL. She doesn't usually know that these products have the same ingredients used in the toothache medicines and products for sore gums. Most of these products will work a lot better if you apply these products directly to the sore gums and teeth. The only exception to this is teething pain, since the pain in that case is coming from within the gum itself.

In cutting teeth, however, the pain comes from within the gum; it's actually caused by the cutting action of the tooth working its way to the surface of the gum. Most of these products contain a deadening ingredient, the most common being BENZOCAINE. It will provide some temporary relief, but don't expect too much help from these products. (While you're at the drugstore you might want to pick up some ear plugs as well.)

Usually in the infant area of the drugstore where you find the other products, you will also notice teething rings. Some contain a GEL that you can place in the ice box and cool. When your baby chews on them, the cooling effect will often help to soothe his or her gums. The other kinds of teething rings are made of RUBBER or LATEX and they work pretty well too; by biting on these rings the child helps cut down on the pain associated with teething. You can also use your finger to gently massage the irritated gum area. But be careful; if there are any teeth around the area you're massaging, you could wind up regretting it.

If you do decide to use one of the gel types, and if your child has some teeth already, be sure he doesn't bite through the teething ring and swallow the gel. The gel is made of safe material, but it could upset the child's stomach.

If you decide to use one of the teething lotions, remember that they sometimes cause ALLERGIC REACTIONS. If your child develops a RASH, or the lotion seems to irritate the gums more, stop using it and ask your doctor's advice. Teething children require time and patience, and that is something that you just do not find on a drugstore shelf.

27
INSULIN

More and more people every year are diagnosed as being DIABETIC. Some cases can be controlled by diet alone. Others may require an oral prescription medicine, while still others must rely on daily injections of INSULIN for the rest of their lives. There are several different kinds of insulin available, and each one works a little differently in the body. The different sorts are usually indicated by differently colored boxes. So always be sure that you buy the right one for you.

Insulin is available in three strengths: U-40, U-80, and U-100. This means that there are, respectively, 40 units of insulin in each cubic centimeter, 80 units, and 100 units. Lately some strengths of insulin have become harder to find, especially the U-40 and U-80 strengths. That is because the large manufacturers are in the process of making only one strength available, the U-100. This is causing a lot of confusion in the minds of people who use insulin; remember that the U-100 solution is the same kind of insulin as the others, only it is more concentrated. This means that you do not have to inject yourself with as much insulin each time; therefore, a bottle will last longer. There is no real savings in buying the U-100 and you will have to use the U-100 syringes and needles.

With the number of diabetics growing each year, there has been great concern that our supplies of insulin would become inadequate at some time in the future, since insulin is made from the pancreas glands of cattle and hogs. But recently the Eli Lilly Company, who were pioneers in the development of insulin, have introduced the first synthetic insulin. The product is now being tested on human volunteers and the results are very favorable. As a matter of fact we will probably see this product on the market in the very near future, as Eli Lilly Company is building a new facility strictly for the production of synthetic insulin. This is good news for those who rely on daily injections to maintain their health and lead normal lives.

Diabetics sometimes ask the pharmacist if there are syringes that are easier to read than others, since diabetics' eyesight is typically not very strong. Ask your pharmacist about a magnifying glass that is available from the Sherwood Company, the makers of **MONOJECT** syringes and needles, and that snaps right onto the syringe. It magnifies the numbers so that they are easy to read when you are drawing up your insulin. If your pharmacist can't order one for you, check with your local Diabetes Association and see if they can help you.

Diabetics also should check their urine periodically to make sure that the insulin is keeping the diabetes under control. Because diabetes is hereditary, it might be a good idea to include other members of your family in your urine-testing program.

Always stay in close contact with your doctor, and report any unusual problems that develop. Make sure when you are buying over-the-counter or other products that they do not contain sugar. Many of them do, to make the product taste better. Ask for your pharmacist's help in selecting a safe and effective product.

Foot care is also very important for diabetics since leg and foot circulation is often poor, increasing the chance of infection. Be extremely careful when using corn and callus removers, for example. This also means no bathroom surgery, such as cutting out ingrown toe nails, or trimming calluses. Check with your doctor first. In these cases his help is very valuable.

28
LAXATIVES

Everyone has needed a laxative at one time or another. Laxatives work by stimulating movement of the intestine, which forces out waste material. The most frequent users of laxatives are elderly people because, unfortunately, the older we get the less active we become. Even our bodily functions slow down. As the saying goes, you can tell you are getting older when you start listening to laxative commercials. Laxatives are used by people to give them regularity in their bowel movements. The problem is, regularity is vaguely defined. One study showed that the range of bowel movement frequency in humans is from three times per day to three times per week. So constipation cannot be defined solely in terms of the number of bowel movements in any given period.

Constipation can be caused by a variety of conditions:

- environmental changes
- failure to acquire a regular habit
- faulty eating habits
- mental stress
- taking certain prescription drugs
- laxative abuse

If you suffer from constipation, try to figure out what might be causing your problem. When you take laxatives routinely, for instance, they may cause laxative dependency. That means that your intestine becomes very lazy and needs laxatives to stimulate each movement. Constipation can often be relieved by eating a high-fiber diet, plentiful liquid consumption, and regular exercise. When we were kids and had a constipation problem, we were always told to drink a warm glass of water. Perhaps our water was piped in from Mexico, but it sure did the trick. Of course, if it didn't, Mom always had the old stand-by, FLETCHERS CASTORIA. One teaspoonful of that before you went to bed and you definitely would not need an alarm clock to get you up in the morning. I guess laxatives will always remind me of when I worked in a drugstore as a student. I remember the pharmacist recommending CITRATE OF MAGNESIA, or, as we called it "Liquid Can Opener." One evening while he was out eating supper, an elderly gentleman came into the store. When I asked if I could help him he said that he was constipated and what would be a good laxative. I realized that this was my chance to act like a pharmacist, so I told him to drink a bottle of Citrate of Magnesia before he went to bed. (That's how I remembered taking a laxative when I was a kid.) The next day he came into the drugstore mad as a hornet. He said he drank down the bottle and went to bed. About four hours later all hell broke loose. It is important to know what you want your laxative to do for you, because not only do laxatives work differently, but they also work at different times.

STIMULANT LAXATIVES

Stimulant laxatives work by irritating the lining of the intestines, which in turn irritates the nerves that cause the intestinal muscles to move and causes bowel movement. Stimulant laxatives are contraindicated with ABDOMINAL

PAIN, NAUSEA, or VOMITING; these are symptoms of APPEN-DICITIS. Stimulant laxatives are effective but should be used cautiously and are not recommended for routine use by people with simple constipation. They should never be used for longer than one week of regular treatment, nor should you exceed the recommended dosage. Among the ingredients most commonly used in stimulant laxatives is BISACODYL, which is available in tablets and suppository form. The tablets usually work in six to ten hours. The rectal suppositories work in 15 to 60 minutes. It is an ingredient found in DULCOLAX. PHENOLPHTHAEIN is another ingredient found in some stimulant laxatives such as EX-LAX, FEEN-A-MINT, and ALOPHEN and usually works in six to eight hours. ALOE, DANTHRON, CASCARA, and SENNA usually work in eight to twelve hours, or sometimes may require up to 24 hours to work. They can be found in CARTERS LIT-TLE PILLS, DORBANE, DOXIDAN, FLETCHER'S CASTORIA, and GENTLAX.

When you buy a laxative product, read the label. If you see any one of these ingredients you will not only know that it is a stimulant laxative, but also how soon you can expect relief.

STOOL SOFTENERS OR LUBRICANTS

MINERAL OIL and certain digestible plant oils, for example, OLIVE OIL, soften fecal contents by coating them with oil, making it easier to pass them. Using mineral oil as a laxative can cause absorption of the oil-soluble vitamins A and D from our bodies. If you are taking oil-soluble vitamins such as A, D, E, and K at the same time as mineral oil, the vitamins will not be absorbed into your body. They will instead be absorbed into the oil, and then eliminated from your body. Prolonged use of these products may cause deficiencies in these vitamins. Mineral oil should not be taken with meals because it may delay the emptying of the stomach. If large doses are taken, it may lubricate the intestine to the point of causing ANAL LEAKAGE, which could lead to anal ITCHING or HEMORRHOIDS.

These products are mainly designed to soften stools. It is probably better to use an ingredient called DIOCTYL SODIUM SULFOSUCCINATE, found in a product called COLACE, if you are looking for a stool softener rather than a laxative.

SALINE LAXATIVES

Saline laxatives are mainly used for immediate evacuation of the bowel before X-rays, tests, or surgery. These products should never by used for long-term treatment of constipation. The active ingredients in saline laxatives are either MAGNESIUM SULFATE (EPSOM SALTS) or MAGNESIUM CITRATE. They usually work in about three to five hours. Products containing MAGNESIUM should not be used by people with KIDNEY DISEASE.

ENEMAS

Enemas are normally used to prepare patients for surgery, child delivery, and X-ray examination. But occasionally they are used in cases of constipation. An enema works in two to fifteen minutes. The most commonly used is FLEET ENEMA. Care should be taken when administering enemas, since a misdirected or inadequately lubricated nozzle could cause severe irritation to the anal canal.

SUPPOSITORIES

GLYCERIN SUPPOSITORIES have been an old stand-by for infants and adults for years. Inserted rectally, they have an irritant effect and usually produce results in 15 to 60 minutes. Aside from the inconvenience of using a suppository, side effects are minimal.

BULK-PRODUCING LAXATIVES

These laxatives are probably the best choice for simple constipation. DIALOSE and HYDROLOSE contain an ingredient called METHYLCELLULOSE and are available in either powder or capsule form. When these products get into the intestine, they absorb water and swell. This gives the intestine a natural feeling of fullness, which in turn stimulates movement. They are usually effective in 12 to 24 hours, but sometimes may require as long as three days. If you need a laxative that works fast, these products won't do the job. Bulk-producing laxatives may combine with certain drugs, such as the SALICYLATES found in some pain-relievers, and should not be taken together, because they could cause these drugs not to be absorbed into the body properly. Some bulk-producing laxatives (like METAMUCIL and EFFERSYL-LIUM) contain PSYLLIUM, which in combination with the SALICYLATES speeds up movement in the gut, causing the drugs to be passed out more quickly and decreasing absorption.

Remember, regular use of most laxatives, especially the stimulant type, can cause LAXATIVE DEPENDENCY. Excessive use can cause DIARRHEA and VOMITING, which could lead to serious problems.

29

LICE

LICE INFESTATION

Lice are parasites believed to commonly affect humans. There are three types of lice: head lice, body lice, and pubic lice. LICE INFESTATION is a condition that must be recognized and treated as soon as possible. It may exist in people of all ages and social levels; no one is immune. Lice are easily transmitted from person to person by sharing personal articles, such as hats, hair ribbons, combs, towels, and bedding, and by physical contact.

HEAD LICE

Infestation by head lice is more common in children but may also occur in adults. As a matter of fact sometimes schools are closed because of an outbreak of lice that spreads in epidemic proportions. Any part of the scalp may be affected. The ITCHING is often severe. You may notice PUSTULES, BLEEDING areas on the scalp, and matting of the hair. It is important to check your children's hair periodically; the lice can be seen on the scalp, or you may notice small, white sticky eggs on the hair itself.

BODY LICE

These organisms mainly live on the clothing and visit the skin only to feed. The eggs may also be found on the hairs of the affected region.

PUBIC LICE

Pubic lice are more commonly called "crabs," because the organism has long tentacles and resembles a crab. These lice are very noticeable and attach themselves to the skin, usually at the point of emergence of a hair. Infestation is more common in men than in women. The lice are transmitted during sexual activity.

TREATMENT

Lice can be treated with a variety of over-the-counter products such as **RID, CUPREX,** or **A-200 PYRINATE.** You apply them undiluted to the infested areas, such as hair and scalp, until entirely wet. *Do not use on eye lashes or eyebrows.* Allow the solution to remain on the area for ten minutes, no longer, since this is sufficient to kill lice and their eggs. Wash hair thoroughly with warm water and soap or shampoo, then dry the area. Comb the hair thoroughly with a fine-tooth comb. Some products, such as **RID,** provide you with a comb. The combing removes dead lice and eggs. Do not exceed two consecutive applications in 24 hours, because the chemicals may irritate the skin. When using these products avoid getting them in your eyes. The products may be used on children. After you have rid yourself of the lice, here are preventative steps to follow:

- Inspect all family members daily, for at least two weeks, and if they do become infested start the treatment again.

- Sterilize all personal clothing, bed clothes, and bedding of the infested person in hot water, at least 130°F., or by dry cleaning.
- Thoroughly wash all personal articles such as combs, brushes, etc., in hot water (130°F.) for 20 minutes.

Since there really is no immunity from lice, personal cleanliness and avoiding infested persons and their bedding and clothes will aid in preventing infestation. These additional steps are important in order to cut down the chances of infestation:

- Completely change undergarments, clothes, and night wear daily. Wash them in hot water (130°F.).
- Scrub toilet seats and vacuum upholstered furniture, rugs, and floors frequently.
- Tell children not to use borrowed combs or brushes or to wear anyone else's clothes.
- Inspect family members periodically for new lice infestation. If a new outbreak is spotted, don't waste time—begin treatment immediately.

30

LINIMENTS AND MUSCLE RUBS

It is said that physical exercise is good for the mind and the soul. The only problem with strenuous physical activity is that it causes SORE MUSCLES. Soreness may also be due, not to strenuous physical activity, but simply doing something you're not used to. As a matter of fact, since the jogging craze started, the sale of liniments has gone up, especially among people who started running for the first time. One man who came into the drugstore was so sore, he said it hurt when he swallowed.

It seems that each liniment product, such as **ABSORBINE JR., HEET, MINIT-RUB,** and many more, has its version of the claim to give "temporary relief of minor muscular aches and pains resulting from over-exertion and fatigue." Some make the promotional claim that "It actually treats the cause of sore, tired muscles," or "penetrates deep into the skin." These claims usually cause confusion in the minds of the people buying them.

Muscle rubs are available in many forms: ointments, creams, liniments, and lotions. These products contain a variety of different ingredients, but they usually also contain the same few basic ones. The most common ingredients found in liniments are irritants to the skin, such as **METHYL**

SALICYLATE (OIL OF WINTERGREEN), MENTHOL, CAM-
PHOR, and EUCALYPTUS, and are known as "counter-irritants." Counter-irritants are applied locally to produce a
mild local reaction and to increase circulation in the sore
area. They are applied to the skin wherever the pain is
experienced.

Pain is only as intense as it is perceived to be; therefore,
when you apply a substance that produces irritation, that
sensation crowds out the experience of the pain around it—
a kind of mind-over-matter treatment. So look at the ingredients in the liniments or rubs you are about to buy and
know how they will work for you: METHYL SALICYLATE is
probably the most widely used counter-irritant. When it is
rubbed on the skin, it produces mild irritation, and it is
absorbed into the skin to an appreciable extent. The range
of effective concentrations of methyl salicylate is 10–60 percent. Methyl salicylate has a very pleasant odor and taste,
similar to candy, which may attract children. *Actually as little as one teaspoonful may be fatal.* So if you use products
containing methyl salicylate, put them in a place completely
out of the reach of children. CAMPHOR is found in many
muscle rubs because it causes redness of skin. It also has a
local anesthetic effect. MENTHOL is used in muscle rubs
because it has a mild anesthetic effect and produces a feeling
of coolness. TURPENTINE OIL has been used for a number
of years as a counter-irritant. It does work fairly well in a
concentration of 10–50 percent. However, be careful if you
do use this compound since it could cause blistering of the
skin.

Muscle rubs are available in different forms. Liniments
have alcohol bases and penetrate deeper into the skin.
Lotions, creams, and ointments stay on the skin much
longer, giving you a continuous release of medication.
When applying a rub, keep the following in mind:

- Use only externally, on skin that is not broken.
- Do not apply to eyes, mucous membranes, abnor-
  mally sensitive skin, or skin that is already
  irritated.

- Discontinue using if excessive skin irritation develops.
- If pain persists longer than ten days or if extreme redness is present, call your doctor.
- Check with your doctor before using these products on children under twelve years of age.
- After applying these products, do not cover or tightly bind the treated area.
- If you are planning to use a heating pad or other form of heat treatment, do not use it in combination with a muscle rub. The two together could cause a severe burn to the skin.

HEAT LAMPS

Many people buy heat lamps to relieve muscle pain and soreness. Heat lamps provide warmth and can temporarily relieve aches and pains. However, do not be confused when you shop for them; they are usually found with the sunlamps and there is a difference. Heat lamps generate infrared light. When using an infrared lamp, wear goggles during long sessions to prevent the moisture in the eyes from drying out.

SUNLAMPS

Sunlamps give off ultraviolet light and are mainly used by people who want to look tan all year long. If you use one yourself, remember never to use a sunlamp without a timer. If the timer does not have an automatic shut-off device, make sure it has an alarm loud enough to wake you in case you fall asleep. Always use ultraviolet-filtering goggles to protect your eyes when using a sunlamp. Be aware also that a hot shower or sauna session just before using a sunlamp can leave you more sensitive than usual to ultraviolet light. If you have sensitive skin to begin with, be sure to protect your lips, because the light may make them dry and crack.

A lip sunscreen will also minimize the risk of developing LIP CANCER from repeated exposure to ultraviolet light.

MASSAGE PRODUCTS

There are now available in most drugstores a variety of appliances to massage sore muscles. Products such as back massagers are actually pads that you unfold and place in a chair or lay out flat on your bed. When plugged in they vibrate, which increases circulation to the muscle and helps to heal it.

If these appliances don't appeal to you, you might want to try one of the hand massagers. Some are available in a Swedish design that attaches to the palm of your hand. Simply massage the sore muscles with the hand that holds the massager. Once again, the vibrating action will speed up healing by increasing the circulation. By the way, if you like a warm massage, these products are also made with heat elements, which produce warmth as you massage the muscles.

Massage products may be used with liniments and muscle rubs; they increase the penetration of the analgesics to help heal those sore, aching muscles. In addition to its other effects, a massage is likely to make you feel relaxed, especially if you are tense, causing the muscles tighten up.

DMSO

This is an industrial solvent that has become very popular recently; it is seen as a cure-all for everything from MUSCLE ACHES to ARTHRITIS. **DMSO** stands for **DIMETHYL SULFOXIDE,** a chemical solvent first found to have medicinal properties when workers, using it to de-grease the Alaskan pipeline, noticed that if they had BRUISES or ACHES or pains, DMSO coming into contact with the affected area helped to make the pain go away. The F.D.A. started testing DMSO, but the tests were halted because the chemical was found to cause eye problems. However, since these tests were done on non-primate animals, there was no proof that this would happen in humans. Tests on DMSO resumed, only this time they were done on healthy human volunteers in a controlled study. Simultaneously, companies all around the country began selling it to people, making claims that were not proven. Since the sale of DMSO is illegal in many states, people began going to border states to buy it, often getting inferior products. Some products contained traces of prescription drugs such as CORTISONE. At present, the safest course of action is to await the outcome of the test results that are currently being conducted to see just what problems DMSO will effectively treat. As of right now, we do know that it has some benefits, mainly with soft tissue injuries such as MUSCLE SPRAINS and STRAINS. Tests have also shown that the sooner you apply DMSO to an injury, the better the results. However, many people who use DMSO for the treatment of ARTHRITIS have not received the relief they expected. It is possible, based on available scientific evidence, that DMSO will become one of the standard treatments for certain types of muscle injuries, and we may very well see it on the drugstore shelves right next to the BEN GAY, ABSORBINE JR., and other muscle rubs. The tests being conducted now will show exactly what DMSO will treat at what concentration without serious side effects.

You can help to get this product approved for general use by using DMSO under your doctor's care. He can then report to the F.D.A. and contribute to the growing body of information. After all, we all want to be sure that the products we use are safe.

31

MOUTHWASHES

Next to toothbrushes and toothpastes, the most commonly used over-the-counter dental products are mouthwashes. According to many of the advertisements "bad breath" is a major cause of social unpopularity. Bad breath is generally caused by the presence of bacteria in the mouth. One's breath is usually at its worst upon waking; that is because bacteria grow in the mouth when it is inactive while we are sleeping. Usually within an hour or so after we wake up, the breath returns to normal. Bad breath is also sometimes caused by dyspepsia or other digestive disorders.

The ideal mouthwash should contain a high antiseptic concentration to rapidly kill bacteria in the mouth. Unfortunately, such a dose may be either very irritating to the tissues inside the mouth, or poisonous if swallowed.

Mouthwashes are usually grouped into two types: those that are cosmetic and those that have ingredients to treat a sore throat. SCOPE, LISTERMINT, and LISTERINE, among others, are intended to freshen your breath temporarily. However, say that you have eaten a meal containing onions or garlic. You may gargle with one of these mouthwashes, but after the first few minutes will notice a taste of garlic on your breath again. That is because the garlic is in the stomach and not in the mouth. It is absorbed through the walls of the stomach into the bloodstream. As a result, every time you exhale, you have garlic breath. If you want to mask the odor, try using a breath mint. It stays in your mouth and permeates the exhaled air to hide the odor. Some people use a purse spray, but except for the convenience of carrying it around with you, it is effective no longer than a mouthwash. What is more, a small pocket spray costs about $1.50 whereas a pack of mints cost 25¢.

People sometimes use mouthwashes for the wrong reason. Gargling with the cosmetic mouthwashes when you have a SORE THROAT can actually cause your sore throat to become worse. The alcohol contained in these products evaporates from the throat, drying it out and causing further irritation. For a sore throat, gargle several times a day with lukewarm salt water: one teaspoonful of salt in an eight-ounce glass of warm water. (Too much salt will also irritate the throat.) If you are running a fever along with the sore throat, call your doctor; it may be a sign of infection.

However, some mouthwashes are intended to treat a sore throat. Products such as CHLORASEPTIC and CEPASTAT contain an ingredient called PHENOL, which is a deadening ingredient. These products numb the throat, mouth, and tongue. The problem with using them is that you can't tell if your sore throat is getting better or worse. If you are already treating your infection with antibiotics, these mouthwashes can give you relief during the course of your illness. They are also available in pocket sprays and lozenges.

32
PAIN RELIEVERS

Pain, ranging from headaches, to sore muscles, to arthritis, is something we all suffer from at one time or another. Unfortunately, there is no product on the market to prevent pain, only to treat the symptoms once it begins. However, when you see the number of pain-relieving products available at the drugstore, you may develop a pain someplace else, just trying to decide which one to buy. Advertisements stating that nine out of every ten doctors recommend the ingredients in ANACIN only complicate matters. Another way of putting it is that nine out of ten doctors recommend ASPIRIN, which is the main ingredient in ANACIN. Now when you hear that statement you will know to buy any product that has aspirin in it—the cheapest being as effective as the most expensive. However, before buying any sort of pain reliever, ask yourself some very important questions. For example, do you have other symptoms with your pain? Do you have a FEVER? How high is it and how long have you had it? Are you ALLERGIC to aspirin? Do you have ASTHMA, and are you taking prescription drugs? Do you suffer any STOMACH DISORDERS?

Even though pain is a common experience, some experts say it is a sensation that can be influenced by many factors, such as fatigue, anxiety, and fear. People experience pain differently depending on their personalities. For example, studies show that introverts have a lower threshold for pain than extroverts. Still, whether you are an introvert or extrovert, black or white, male or female, when you have pain, you probably want to get rid of it quickly.

The pain-relieving products found in most drugstores are basically of two types: the aspirin pain relievers and the non-aspirin pain relievers.

ASPIRIN PAIN RELIEVERS

These contain SALICYLATES, which may appear on the package as ACTEYLSALICYLIC ACID and SODIUM SALICYLATE. Some products contain an ingredient called SALICYLAMIDE, which is chemically related to the salicylates and falls under the same guidelines. There are two types of ASPIRIN pain relievers: simple aspirin, like BAYER, and store-brand aspirins or aspirin products that contain other ingredients as well, such as ANACIN, EMPIRIN, or EXCEDRIN. These are most effective in treating mild PAIN and in reducing FEVER and INFLAMMATION. In certain conditions such as MUSCLE STRAIN or ARTHRITIS, reducing inflammation can definitely relieve the pain. However, try to avoid taking aspirin products with the prescription drugs used to treat arthritis. Many of these drugs irritate the stomach; adding aspirin is asking for trouble. If you must use aspirin for additional relief, try to use it in between doses of your prescription drug. Aspirin is also very effective at lowering body temperature; that is why it is so frequently recommended for the fever, aches, and pains of a bout with the FLU.

When children have a fever, many of us grab the old stand-bys that have been used for years, such as ST. JOSEPH'S CHILDREN'S ASPIRIN or BAYER CHEWABLE ASPIRIN. The only problem with these products is that often when children have a fever, they also have an upset stomach. Aspirin's irritating effects may therefore create more of a problem. For kids, then, it may be better to use a non-aspirin pain reliever such as TYLENOL or TEMPRA to reduce fever. However, note that non-aspirin pain relievers do not reduce inflammation; this is especially important for people suffering from arthritis and muscle strain.

If you get relief from aspirin for various problems, but it upsets your stomach, you may want to try a buffered aspirin product such as BUFFERIN or ASCRIPTIN. They contain ingredients to protect the stomach lining while the aspirin is dissolving. People who suffer from chronic stomach problems like ULCERS may want to use an enteric-coated aspirin such as ECOTRIN or A.S.A. ENSEALS (*enteric-coated* means that they dissolve in the intestine rather than the stomach). But use caution with these products, too. If you have any sort of intestinal problem, these products should be avoided.

Aspirin is probably one of the best products on the market for relief from various forms of discomfort. Since most of us keep it on hand, it is important to know that aspirin can go bad. One way to judge is to take the cap off the bottle and smell the tablets. If they smell like vinegar, chances are that the product is no longer effective. Stale aspirin may also upset the stomach more, because one of the break-down by-products of aspirin is ACETIC ACID (vinegar).

One question often asked is what brand of aspirin is best? If you watch the countless television commercials about different aspirin products, you will really be confused. For example, one commercial shows us that most products contain only 325 mg. of aspirin per tablet and concludes that the product with 400 mg. of aspirin is stronger and better. However, both release aspirin into the bloodstream equally quickly, and for most people, 325 mg. relieves discomfort as well as 400 mg. My advice is to buy the store brand; it is almost always cheaper. After all, aspirin is aspirin. Many people assume that since it is so much cheaper and looks unfamiliar, it can't be as good as the highly advertised products. Wrong! Years ago when I worked at a large hospital pharmacy in St. Louis, patients would often receive a box of aspirin when they were discharged from the hospital. Believe you me, when we bought aspirin for the hospital it was not one of the highly advertised brands; we bought it in drums. And people would come back to the hospital to buy more, because they thought that the aspirin they bought in the drugstore wasn't as good. Aspirin is aspirin.

No matter what brand of aspirin you buy, there are a few things to keep in mind. If you suffer from any type of stomach disorder, avoid it. Pregnant women also should try to avoid aspirin as much as possible, especially in the latter stages of pregnancy; because aspirin is an anti-coagulant, it can cause excessive bleeding before and after delivery.

Aspirin also causes ALLERGIC REACTIONS in some people. One type causes SHORTNESS OF BREATH or asthmalike symptoms. The other causes skin reactions, such as REDNESS, SWELLING, and HIVES. So if you suffer from asthma, or chronic hives, you will want to be extremely careful when using aspirin products.

Aspirin also interacts with some prescription drugs. Aspirin has the ability to keep the blood thin—that is, to reduce its tendency to clot. As a matter of fact scientists are now testing aspirin, trying to find out whether it may be effective in preventing a stroke or heart attack because of this unique feature. However, people taking other blood-thinning prescription drugs, such as COUMADIN and DICUMAROL, should try to avoid combining them with aspirin. The two together could thin the blood to the point of causing hemorrhaging. If you do take the both and notice bruising, or reddish-colored urine, *report it to your doctor immediately*.

Aspirin may also counteract medicines containing VITAMIN K. Vitamin K is given to people to cause their blood to clot, while aspirin reduces blood clots.

Some people taking oral medicines for DIABETES should be careful about aspirin. Those taking DIABINESE and ORINASE along with aspirin may develop lower blood sugar levels. Report any unusual signs to your doctor.

Anti-inflammatory prescription drugs, such as INDOCIN, BUTAZOLIDIN, or MOTRIN, should not be combined with aspirin because they can cause stomach ulcers.

Two prescription drugs used to treat GOUT are PROBEN-ECID (BENEMID) and SULFINPYRAZONE (ANTURANE). When combined with aspirin, they could precipitate a gouty attack, or KIDNEY-STONE formation. So if you use aspirin often or occasionally, before you take it along with a prescription drug, check with your pharmacist or doctor to make sure it is safe.

Some of the common side effect of taking too much aspirin are DIZZINESS, RINGING in the ears, difficulty in HEARING, NAUSEA, VOMITING, and DIARRHEA. Very high dosages may cause you to develop incoherent speech, DELIRIUM, or HALLUCINATIONS. And like any other drug, if enough is taken it will cause death. The emergency treatment for aspirin poisoning is to delay emptying of the stomach. If the person is conscious this can be done by drinking two glasses of milk to slow down the absorption of the drug by coating the stomach. You can also give ACTIVATED CHARCOAL.

Vomiting should be induced, by using SYRUP OF IPECAC, or anything else that will cause a person to vomit. However, syrup of Ipecac is not effective in combination with activated charcoal. If you want more information on these drugs, turn to Chapter 34, *Poison Prevention*.

NON-ASPIRIN PAIN RELIEVERS

The most common non-aspirin pain reliever available is ACETAMINOPHEN which is found in TYLENOL, DATRIL, and TEMPRA, as well as in store brands. This drug is effective against NEURALGIA and PAIN in the muscles or bones. It also reduces fever, usually in about 30 minutes after it is taken, and produces its peak effect in two to four hours. The main advantage of the non-aspirin products over aspirin is that there is less irritation to the stomach and so they would be better suited for persons suffering from chronic stomach problems. However, they do not relieve INFLAMMATION as aspirin does, so they are not beneficial to the person suffering from ARTHRITIS or another inflammatory condition.

Because it lacks many side effects produced by aspirin, acetaminophen is gaining popularity in this country as the common household pain reliever. However, there is growing concern about the public's lack of awareness of acetaminophen's toxicity. Acetaminophen has been shown to be harmful to the LIVER, where the drug is broken down and destroyed. However, this problem only occurs when very high doses are taken. Eight 500 mg. capsules or tablets taken daily does not cause any apparent harm, but at twelve to fourteen 500-mg. doses, toxic reactions can occur—VOMITING within a few hours, loss of APPETITE, NAUSEA, and STOMACH PAIN within 24 hours. There is also evidence of liver damage and jaundice within two to four days. Emergency first aid is the same as for aspirin; use milk or activated charcoal to slow down absorption into the system. Also induce vomiting with SYRUP OF IPECAC. Obviously, people with chronic liver conditions, or weakened livers from excessive drinking, must be careful when using ACETAMINOPHEN; it may speed up deterioration of the liver. If you don't know for sure, check with your doctor before buying it.

One often sees the words "extra strength" on the packages of pain relief products. Such products are usually combinations of several pain-relieving ingredients and may include ASPIRIN, SALICYLAMIDE, and ACETAMINOPHEN. Because the total of pain-relieving ingredients may be more than 325 mg. (5 grams), the implication is that these products are stronger and more effective. Combinations of ingredients have not been proven to be more effective than an equal amount of an individual ingredient. Some products making this claim simply contain an increased dosage of the same ingredient, for example, TYLENOL and TYLENOL EXTRA-STRENGTH. The way I look at it is this: If you are using one plain TYLENOL tablet and it gives you relief, why buy the more expensive extra-strength product? But if you normally take two tablets at a time, you might save money and get the same relief by taking one of the extra-strength tablets or capsules. Let common sense be your guide.

In spite of the huge variety of products available to consumers there are really only a few pain relievers. Knowing how these ingredients work and what to avoid makes the choice a lot simpler.

33

PET SUPPLIES

Nowadays most drugstores have a section dedicated to pets. After all, most people love their pets almost as much as they love their children. Aside from giving him rawhide bones, flea collars, and shampoos, there are also things you can do at home to treat your pet during illness. Obviously, some of these tips are only temporary measures, until you can get your pet to the vet.

If your pet's eyes are WATERY, wash them with milk rather than water because milk is closer to their tearfilm. Or you may use any ordinary eye wash you have around the house.

ASPIRIN is safe to give to your dog occasionally. However, try to use BUFFERED ASPIRIN. Simple aspirin may cause irritation to the stomach and possibly cause your dog to vomit. Do not give your dog more than one adult 5-grain aspirin for 40 to 50 pounds of body weight every twelve hours, because it stays in their system longer than in humans'. Never give aspirin to cats: Because of the long excretion time, a toxic build-up in the body could occur.

If your dog or cat has gotten into a poisonous product, be sure to save the container for the vet's information. Make him vomit by giving him HYDROGEN PEROXIDE, SYRUP OF IPECAC, or SALT WATER, unless the poison is an ACID or

ALKALI. If it is an acid, give a solution of baking soda (SODIUM BICARBONATE). If it is an alkali, give lemon juice or milk. Dogs have been known to eat anti-freeze. If this happens, give gin or vodka until the dog is slightly drunk. Then *rush* him to the vet.

Suppose your pet gets paint, tar, or asphalt on his coat. Never use paint remover or kerosene! Trim away as much of the coating as possible and soak the remaining fur in vegetable oil for one hour or overnight, then shampoo it. If you have no dog shampoo handy, use JOY detergent; it is less irritating to the skin than other detergents. If your pet has dry skin apply diluted ALPHA KERI BATH OIL. Sometimes pets get sprayed by skunks during a romp in the woods. Use tomato juice to remove the smell.

Following are other common problems and treatments:

- Coughing: Use a children's cough syrup (without aspirin).
- Simple diarrhea: Give KAOPECTATE or PEPTO BISMOL. Start with several tablespoonfuls every few hours.
- Insect stings: Apply a paste of baking soda.
- Burns: Soak in cold water, then apply a bland ointment. *Do not use butter.*
- Mild constipation: Give MILK OF MAGNESIA, but beware of CASTOR OIL.

However, it is safe to place one drop of castor oil in the eye to prevent soap from getting into the animal's eyes while bathing. These are a few of the home remedies for various problems your pet develops. Remember, though, to check with your vet in the specific instance, just to be sure.

People often feel that pet products bought in the drugstore are safe. However, always read carefully the instructions on the product you are buying and follow them to the letter. Individuals (animal or human) may be ALLERGIC to certain ingredients, so watch for symptoms when administering a new product.

Three of the most common pet products are:

- **FLEA COLLARS:** When putting one on your pet, allow two fingers between the collar and the neck. Do not leave the end long because your pet may chew on it. Before putting on the flea collar, leave it out in the air for 24 hours and do not allow it to get wet.
- **WORM MEDICINE:** Before using any of the worm medicines, have the stool of your pet checked by a vet, because different worms require different treatments. Never give worm medicine to a sick dog. Also, these products do not work prophylactically. Therefore, do not give once a month for prevention or "just in case."
- **PET SHAMPOOS:** Many of these products are fine for normal use, but be sure to rinse the soap out thoroughly. Residues left behind could irritate the skin. Do not bathe your pet too often—in fact the less, the better, unless your pet has a condition for which your vet is treating him. If your pet has a skin condition be sure to check with your vet first; he or she may advise you to use a special shampoo.

Keep all these things in mind and your pet will stay healthy, and like as not, will not mind going out in the bitter cold to get your morning newspaper.

34

POISON PREVENTION

Each year, emergency rooms around the country see thousands of children who accidentally eat or drink a poisonous product around the house. If only parents had taken the necessary steps in advance, they might have prevented a serious, or even fatal, poisoning. So let us take a look at three areas of the home where most accidental poisonings occur.

BASEMENT OR GARAGE

This is the area of the house where we store products such as GASOLINE, CHARCOAL LIGHTER, TURPENTINE, and INSECTICIDES. If you do have such products on hand, always make sure to keep them in their original containers, tightly capped. If possible use a safety closure cap. When you are not using these products, keep them well out of the reach of children. If you are using these products, never keep them in soda bottles, cups, or glasses; kids associate these things with eating and drinking. Also, when you are using these products, do not let them out of your sight, even if that means carrying them with you if you have to answer

the phone, or if you talk to a neighbor. Kids act fast, and so
do poisons.

UNDER THE KITCHEN SINK

This is usually the area of the home where we store products such as drain openers, oven cleaners, and other household cleaners. Unfortunately, this area is easy for the child
to reach. If you must store these products under your sink,
be sure to store them in their original containers, since most
products show an antidote on the package. Often people
want to know how they can tell if their child has taken one
of these products. Reactions vary depending on the product.
The child may VOMIT or appear SLUGGISH and TIRED for no
apparent reason. You may see a residue around the mouth
and teeth of the child, or see that the contents of the package are drastically reduced.

The important thing is to act fast, even if you only suspect that your child has gotten into a particular package.
Check the container to see if there is an antidote on the
package. Keep the poison control center phone number for
your community posted with your other emergency numbers. The number will put you in touch with dedicated individuals who are standing by 24 hours a day to provide you
with life-saving information. Many poison control centers
across the country distribute Mr. Yuk stickers on request.
The stickers show a picture of an ugly face. Place them on
all products that may be harmful, and instruct the children
to stay away from those products that have the sticker on
them.

BATHROOM MEDICINE CABINET

This is the area of the home where most accidental poisonings occur. As a matter of fact, it is not the best place to
keep your medicine; a child may go into the bathroom and

lock the door behind him, and you will have trouble getting to that child fast enough. In addition, many medicines are affected by heat and moisture, which often build up in a bathroom. If you do keep your medicine there, always store it in its original container, with a child-proof lid. If you buy your medicines with the plain cap because they are easier to open and you don't have any small children, remember that children sometimes come over to visit. If they do, be sure to move your medicine to a place of safety, out of their reach. Also, clean out the medicine cabinet periodically and get rid of old or unused medicines. Do this by dumping the contents into the toilet and flushing them away. If you get up during the night to take something, be sure to turn on the light so that you can see what you are taking.

The next thing you can do is to look around your house and correct any problem areas. That one small step may prevent an accidental poisoning from happening to you or any member of your family.

SYRUP OF IPECAC

The antidotes on most packages tell you to induce VOM-ITING, although there are products for which vomiting is not prescribed. In any case, to cause vomiting is usually a lot easier said than done. Some people drink a soapy solution, others stick something down the throat to cause gagging and vomiting. However, there is a product in your corner drugstore that is almost 100 percent effective. It is called SYRUP OF IPECAC. Syrup of Ipecac is safe and effective. Give children one tablespoonful followed by 8 ounces of water. Adults take two tablespoonfuls and 8 ounces to a pint of water. It is very important to drink water after a dose of Ipecac, because it helps the drug to be absorbed more quickly. Vomiting usually occurs in about 15 to 20 minutes. If it does not, repeat the dosage.

Syrup of Ipecac should be a permanent fixture in any home that has kids. It could save a life.

35

PREGNANCY AND OVER-THE-COUNTER DRUGS

At a time when there are many prescription and over-the-counter drugs on the market, researchers are finding that some drugs have a direct effect on fetuses. It is therefore very important to detect pregnancy early and to take the right step to safeguard your health, as well as the health of your unborn child. One method of early detection is the do-it-yourself-at-home pregnancy test kit. These tests are not only accurate, but have also made a lot of rabbits happy.

The benefits of knowing that you are pregnant within a few weeks after conception are boundless. Proper diet, exercise, and prenatal care can be started immediately to ensure a healthy baby. Before the test kits were available, if a woman missed a period she called her doctor. Usually he told her if she missed another period to make an appointment. By the time she got in to see her doctor she was through the first three months or trimester of pregnancy, a critical time for the unborn child. With the home pregnancy test kits you can test yourself to see if you are pregnant seven days after you miss your first period. Quite a difference!

If you do use the home pregnancy test kits, consider these important factors not found on the package instructions:

The test may be taken anywhere from seven to nine days after a missed period; tests taken to prove the accuracy of these products were taken closer to two weeks after a missed period. The test is extremely delicate. Room temperature should not be too high or too low. And the container used to collect the urine should be free from dirt or detergent residue since these could cause a faulty reading. The slightest movement, such as children running through the room or the vibration of a refrigerator or air conditioner can change the reading. Direct sunlight may affect it. If urine is not normal to begin with, the test may not only be inaccurate but may give a positive reading of something other than pregnancy. (It can show up some diseases or certain medications.)

Regardless of the outcome of the pregnancy test reading, you should contact your doctor. There may be other reasons for missing your period that may need medical attention. And the possibility of a misreading exists; if you get a negative reading, the kit directions suggest you try again in another week or so. The kits cost about nine to ten dollars.

Many pregnant women take medication. Estimates indicate that each pregnant woman in this country takes an average of four to five prescription medications, plus over-the-counter drugs, and has an undetermined exposure to potentially toxic substances in food, cosmetics, household chemicals, and the general environment.

The normal rate of birth defects of all kinds is two to three percent. Recently, a study was conducted of 1,369 pregnant women, almost all of whom took at least one prescription drug, and well over half of whom took over-the-counter drugs as well. One-third of the births to the women in the study had some kind of defect. No definite cause was found for this occurrence. However, the study concluded that prescription and over-the-counter drugs should be avoided whenever possible. Unfortunately, in many cases, pregnant women take as many, if not more, drugs than non-pregnant women. These drugs may have adverse affects on the mother and on the fetus.

Among all membrane systems of the body, the placenta is unique; it separates two distinct individuals with differing genetic compositions, physiologic responses, and sensitivities to drugs. The fetus gets nutrients and eliminates waste through the placenta without having to depend on its own immature organs. However, when foreign substances appear in the mother's blood, the placenta does not form a true barrier between mother and fetus. In fact, most drugs that enter the mother's body will also enter the fetus.

A very important period is the first two weeks after conception. During this period, there is no differentiation of cells in the embryo. If enough cells are harmed by a drug, then the embryo will die. No congenital malformations happen at this early stage; it is an "all-or-nothing" situation. During the next one or two months, the organ systems are developing, and this time period is the most critical for the development of abnormalities. After the end of the eighth week, differentiation of the organs is completed. So, the first trimester of pregnancy is the most significant period for the occurrence of deformities and the survival of the fetus. If possible, during the first trimester no medicine of any kind should be taken unless advised by a doctor, including nonprescription drugs for colds, coughs, nervousness, and insomnia. The following are some of the possible adverse effects an unborn child may suffer if the mother takes drugs:

- Antibiotics of the TETRACYCLINE class, which are often prescribed for bacterial infections, may cause permanent discoloration of the child's teeth. QUININE and STREPTOMYCIN may cause deafness.
- Hormones, such as DIETHYLSTIBESTEROL (DES), have been demonstrated to cause vaginal cancer in some young women, as a result of fetal exposure when the mother was administered the drug to prevent miscarriage.
- Although consuming adequate vitamins during pregnancy is very important to both mother and

fetus, excessive amounts can be dangerous. High levels of calcium in the blood and mental retardation may result from excessive amounts of VITAMIN D.

- Large amounts of VITAMIN B-6 and VITAMIN C, although not stored in the body, have been shown to cause withdrawal seizures in the newborn.

- BARBITURATES, taken throughout pregnancy or in the last three months, may cause the infant to be born with an ADDICTION to barbiturates.

- AMPHETAMINES, taken by many women to aid in weight loss, has the potential to cause BIRTH DEFECTS.

- Minor TRANQUILIZERS, such as VALIUM, LIBRIUM, and MILTOWN (MEPROBAMATE), taken during early pregnancy, increase the chance that the baby will be born with a CLEFT LIP or PALATE.

- Aspirin or drugs containing SALICYLATES may prolong pregnancy when taken in the last three months or cause excessive BLEEDING in the mother before and after delivery.

- ALCOHOL is a powerful drug and consuming even one to three ounces a day will probably harm the fetus. Studies show that STILLBIRTHS, PREMATURE BIRTH, MENTAL RETARDATION, and PHYSICAL and BEHAVIORAL PROBLEMS are found in children born to alcoholic mothers.

- Smoking TOBACCO, especially daily, increases the chance that the baby will have a below-normal birth weight.

- Scientists are now looking into the effects of CAFFEINE on the newborn child. Tests show that there may be a link between the consumption of large amounts of caffeine and birth deformities.

- A final hazard is exposure to XRAYS during pregnancy. The cells of the unborn child are dividing rapidly and forming into specialized cells and tissues which are sensitive to radiation. During the earliest weeks of pregnancy, especially avoid X-rays of the abdomen, lower back, pelvis, and hip.

Although a drug may be implicated in the occurrence of birth defects, it is difficult to determine if the drug is the primary culprit. In many instances, the pregnant woman has been exposed to other hazards, such as environmental pollution or diseases that may cause abnormalities. Before a drug is administered to a pregnant woman, the benefits to her must be carefully weighed against the possible harm to the fetus. The majority of drugs consumed by pregnant women are related to effects of pregnancy. These include prenatal vitamins, antacids, mild pain relievers, and laxatives. Most of the agents in these catagories do not cause problems. However there are several drugs in these groups as well as in many others that should be avoided during pregnancy.

ASPIRIN and aspirin-containing products are probably the largest-selling over-the-counter products that should be avoided during pregnancy. If you have a headache, try an ice pack on the head, lie quietly in a dark room, or simply take a walk and get away from the problem that caused the headache in the first place. If these treatments don't work you may use a pain reliever such as TYLENOL or DATRIL, but try to stay away from the SALICYLATES.

For coughs and colds, be careful about the cough syrup you use. Some have alcohol bases. Since alcohol should be avoided in pregnancy, it is obviously a good idea to avoid these cough syrups, such as NYQUIL, as well. Also avoid cough syrups containing CODEINE, such as ROBITUSSIN A-CV, TERPIN HYDRATE AND CODEINE ELIXER, and CHERACOL. If you have a cough and cold, drink a lot of fluids, rest, and keep warm.

If you must use an over-the-counter product, pick one

with a single ingredient and not a combination product, to avoid introducing unnecessary drugs into your and your child's bodies.

Finally, if you are pregnant or even suspect you are, tell your doctor before he writes your prescription, or ask your pharmacist about any medication you are presently taking and about the over-the-counter products you use regularly.

Once the child is born, drugs can cause a problem if you are breast feeding your baby. In recent years there has been a marked upsurge in breast feeding by American mothers. While this trend has some of the elements of faddism, it probably should be welcomed by physicians as a contribution to infant health. There is strong evidence that breast milk contains ANTIBODIES that may help safeguard infants against INFECTION while their own immune systems are maturing.

Despite the evident advantages of this natural method of infant nutrition, one should probably consider the fact that the human animal is no longer living in a natural state. The lactating mother is, or may be, exposed to a host of unnatural substances, including drugs and other active chemicals that may be either ingested deliberately (ALCOHOL, NICOTINE) or absorbed passively from the environment. Some—though by no means all—of these substances pass into the milk in large enough amounts to affect the metabolism of the baby nourished by it. Some—for example, most ANTIHISTAMINES—inhibit lactation. Others may incapacitate the mother to properly care for the infant (MARIJUANA, LSD).

Mild ANALGESICS, including aspirin, ACETAMINOPHEN, and the prescription drug DARVON, are compatible with breast feeding. ERGOT preparations, used to treat MIGRAINES, are not compatible, since they produce VOMITING, DIARRHEA, and other toxic affects in the infant. The only time these drugs should not cause a problem is in the period immediately after birth, when they may be used to control uterine BLEEDING.

Narcotic pain relievers are safe when used in therapeutic doses. Tranquilizers and sedatives should, for the most part, be used with caution or not at all. Barbiturates are very unpredictable. Some seem safe in therapeutic doses, and others probably should be avoided. Most anti-infective drugs are safe for the infant, with the exception of TETRA-CYCLINE, which can permanently stain the child's teeth.

Hormones should be used with caution or not at all. This applies to oral contraceptives, the hormonal content of which can pass into the breast milk, with possible risk to the infant. Many physicians have the mother use an alternative contraceptive method during breast feeding.

Most laxatives are safe. Exceptions are preparations containing CASCARA and ALOE, which can give your baby diarrhea. Some herb teas contain laxative substances that could produce diarrhea in the infant.

NICOTINE should be avoided. Maternal smoking of more than one pack of cigarettes per day can cause RESTLESSNESS, DIARRHEA, and VOMITING and can speed up a baby's hearbeat.

The important thing to keep in mind when breast feeding is that if you are taking a drug, whether prescription or non-prescription, it can often be replaced with a drug that would be more compatible with your baby's system.

36
SHAMPOOS AND HAIR PRODUCTS

The shampoo section of the drugstore has grown by leaps and bounds. As a matter of fact, there are so many products available that you are likely to see not only shelves, but also baskets and barrels full of shampoos. As long as they all work to clean the hair, pick the cheapest product.

Some shampoos say they make the hair shiny, others say they make it more manageable, and they all claim to make you beautiful. Many shampoos are "pH-balanced." But most people don't really know what that means. PH is the measurement of how acidic or alkaline a given thing is. Our skins, hair, scalps, and fingernails are all on the acid side. So you can run into real problems by using shampoos that have soapy bases. Soap is very alkaline. If you don't rinse it all off the scalp, you will get a build-up of alkalinity on the hair. Those deposits of alkalinity can eventually smother and destroy the hair follicle itself.

Therefore, it is probably a good idea to buy a pH-balanced shampoo, since it can actually work in harmony with the skin. Even if you fail to wash it completely out of your hair, you probably won't have serious problems. Pick the one that best suits your pocketbook, since most of the pH-balanced shampoos work in the same way.

Another group of shampoos are those containing protein

and conditioners. These types of shampoos are generally good for the hair, but some people benefit more than others. You are likely to benefit if you are out in the sun a lot, because the sun bleaches the hair fibers and makes them brittle. If you have a job where chemicals or dust are in the air, these may damage the hair. If you have tinted or bleached hair, the natural protein may be stripped out of your hair. In these conditions, it may be best to use a shampoo with protein in it, to replace the protein in your hair. However, be very careful when choosing such a shampoo. Some do not work as well as others. Look for one containing HYDROLIZED ANIMAL PROTEIN. Protein from other sources doesn't do much for the hair. Conditioners work hand-in-hand with the protein in shampoos. Because the conditioners work by coating the hair fibers, they prevent the hair from losing protein and moisture. They also give the hair more body and luster. As with other products, know what you want a shampoo to do for you.

DANDRUFF

If you notice ITCHING and FLAKING regardless of how often you shampoo, you may have DANDRUFF. Dandruff is not a disease but a normal condition like the growth of hair and nails, except that the end product is visible on the scalp as well as on your clothing. It could have a cosmetic and social impact. Dandruff usually appears at puberty when many skin activites are altered, reaches a peak in early adulthood, levels off at middle age, and declines with advancing years. There is no cure for dandruff, only control of the condition. Of course, total removal of the hair will eliminate dandruff. However, that is a pretty drastic solution.

The best way to treat dandruff is by cleaning the hair and scalp frequently, perhaps daily. This should be sufficient to control dandruff, but you may also try one of the dandruff shampoos. One type, SELSUN-BLUE, contains SELENIUM SULFIDE. This ingredient reduces the production of tissue on the scalp and is fairly effective at controlling dandruff. Some products, such as SEBULEX, contain SALICYLIC ACID and SULPHUR. The sulphur helps cut down the production of oil on the scalp and the salicylic acid helps remove the built-up tissue from the scalp. These ingredients also work very well in the treatment of dandruff. Before buying a dandruff shampoo, examine your scalp; there is no INFLAMMATION or REDNESS of the scalp with dandruff. If you do notice redness where the FLAKING is, check with your doctor before using an over-the-counter dandruff shampoo. You may have SEBORRHEA or PSORIASIS, and in that case your doctor will want you to use a specific medicated shampoo to treat your condition. If you do decide to use one of the over-the-counter dandruff shampoos, be sure to follow the directions exactly. Usually after shampooing the hair, you leave the lather on the scalp for about five minutes so that the ingredients can work effectively, rinse it out, and shampoo your hair with your regular shampoo. But be sure to rinse the dandruff shampoo from your scalp thoroughly. If you leave a residue on the hair, it will fall to the scalp and combine with the dandruff to form larger flakes which are even more noticeable.

Some shampoos contain TAR, which advertisers claim is a good treatment for dandruff, but tar is mainly used to treat psoriasis. Let your doctor be the judge. Makers of some dandruff shampoos claim that you can feel your scalp tingle when the shampoo is working. Often these shampoos contain MENTHOL along with other ingredients, and the tingle you feel is nothing more than the cooling effect of the menthol on the scalp. It is doubtful that these products are any more effective than other dandruff shampoos on the market. If you are confused about which one to buy, ask your pharmacist. He will make your selection a lot easier.

BALDNESS

Of course, some people lose more than flakes from their heads. Unfortunately that gradual but increasing loss of hair is called male pattern baldness and it affects many people. This form of baldness is hereditary and is usually caused by a build-up of the male hormone TESTOSTERONE in the scalp, causing an acidic condition that destroys the hair. The reason some hair stays in is because it is under different genetic control than other parts of the scalp. Men often come into the drugstore and ask for a vitamin or hair product to restore their hair. Unfortunately no product can do that. Some products are claimed to promote the growth of hair because they contain female hormones. The only problem is that the hair they produce is usually nothing more than white fuzz. Other products state that 80 percent of the people who use the product experience complete hair regrowth. The people who buy these products and find they don't work are simply told that they fall into the 20 percent failure category. Do not waste your money looking for a miracle. Ways of coping with baldness that do work include hair transplants or hair replacements. If you are losing your hair and you are concerned about it, you might want to check with a qualified hair expert for advice. (My theory is that when God created heads, the ones that didn't turn out right he covered with hair.)

HAIR DYES

There are also a number of products on the market to color the hair. Some of these products can be rinsed out of the hair and others permanently color the hair—in order to get them out, you must wait until the hair grows out.

Always be careful when using hair dyes. They contain chemicals that can burn the eye. If this should happen, flush the eye immediately with water. It might also be helpful to use an eye wash. Be sure to follow the instructions for the hair dye closely; if they tell you to wear rubber gloves, be sure you do. Some hair dyes may cause an allergic reaction of the skin, so it would be a good idea to test the product on a small area of the skin before using it. Also remember that these products are not intended to be used on the eyebrows because of the possibility of burning the eye. It is when you try to take short-cuts that needless accidents can happen. Before you buy a product read the instructions carefully. If it seems confusing, it would probably be to your advantage to have the dyeing done at a hairdresser's.

Other products that may be dangerous are those that gradually darken hair, such as GRECIAN FORMULA. They contain LEAD ACETATE to darken the hair. However, the F.D.A. is now requiring the manufacturers of these products to put a warning on the label that they contain lead. This warning is not there just to decorate the package, even though these products contain only a small amount of lead and absorption through the scalp is poor. If you have any open wounds on the scalp or suffer from a scalp condition such as psoriasis, absorption would be higher.

HAIR BRUSHES

People often want to know what brush to use. The natural-bristle ones are best, as they help to distribute oil throughout the hair. Then again, with today's hair styles, most people want a dry, fluffy look. If you have long hair—that is, over the ears—use a wide-bristle brush. For short hair use a natural-bristle brush. If you notice the brush pulling your hair, it could mean that you need a wider bristle, or that you have damaged hair. Check with your hairdresser. As the saying goes, "Only your hairdresser knows for sure."

HAIR DRYERS

These are now available in many shapes, sizes, and colors, unlike many years ago when you put a plastic hat on your head and dried your hair while you polished your nails or read a magazine. Today's hair dryers are portable, compact, and easy to use. But they can burn or damage the hair.

Try to pick one with a low maximum temperature. A way to check is to turn it on using the hot setting and hold your hand about six inches away from it. If it burns you to the point that you have to pull your hand away, the dryer could hurt your hair. The wattage on the hair dryer does not mean a thing; it is the amount of heat given off that is important. When buying a hair dryer make sure it produces a lot of air movement. The higher the velocity of air it puts out, the better it will be for your hair.

37

SLEEPING AIDS

Nothing is as restful as a good night's sleep, but almost *half* the American population fails to achieve this seemingly simple goal. Some people have trouble falling asleep, others awaken in the middle of the night and cannot go back to sleep. In those situations, it seems that the more one looks at the alarm clock on the night stand, the more one panics, making it almost impossible to get to sleep.

Even though almost half the population has trouble falling asleep, the selection of sleeping aids in the drugstores is rather limited. All of the nonprescription sleeping aids contain an antihistamine, usually either METHAPYRILENE or PYRILAMINE MALEATE. You will find a listing right on the package.

Recently it was reported that the F.D.A. was considering taking these products off the market, because they cause cancerous tumors in laboratory animals. However, the ingredients have not been linked to cancer in humans, which is why the products are still available. Since the time of that report, a new product, called UNISOM and containing a different antihistamine, has been marketed. If you are concerned about the product you are using now, at least there is an alternative.

Perhaps you are wondering what an antihistamine is doing in a product supposed to induce sleep. Remember that antihistamines have the side effect of causing drowsiness, exactly what one needs to sleep. Some products, such as COMPOZ, NERVINE, NYTOL, and SLEEP-EZE, contain nothing but an antihistamine.

Other products contain both an antihistamine and a pain reliever: for example, SOMINEX, QUIET WORLD, and TRANQUIL. These products may be effective if pain is what is keeping you awake in the first place.

Although these products are promoted as being safe and non-habit forming, antihistamines do have side effects, which include DIZZINESS, RINGING in the ears, BLURRED VISION, and DRYNESS of the mouth and throat. Large doses of antihistamines stimulate the central nervous system, resulting in nervousness and irritability. However, the antihistamines used in these products do have a wide margin of safety if you follow the dosage instruction on the package. If these products do not not work for you, check with your doctor: INSOMNIA may be a sign of serious underlying illness, such as ANXIETY or DEPRESSION.

NON-CHEMICAL WAYS TO GET TO SLEEP

If people who have difficulty falling asleep would take the time to figure out what is keeping them awake, they might cure their insomnia without taking anything at all. If you wake up during the night, get out of bed and walk around for a while before trying to go back to sleep. If you have trouble falling asleep, try watching television or reading a book; these activities tire the eyes, often to the point of causing them to close. Some people drink a glass of warm milk, which helps relax them so that they can get to sleep.

Another way of relaxing your body is to soak in a tub of water, as hot as you can stand it. The hot water helps relax the muscles and releases the tension that has built up in them all day. Some people find that physical exercise, followed by a hot shower, will cause them to feel tired and sleepy.

Finally, if you wake up during the night to void fluids, and afterwards cannot get back to sleep, you may want to limit your intake of fluids in the evening from about nine o'clock on. If these suggestions sound too simple, remember that it is often the simple methods that work best.

38
STIMULANTS

How many of us remember staying up late cramming for final exams? It usually meant taking a product like NODOZ or VIVARIN to stay awake and alert. It has been proven that these products do help increase mental alertness when sheer boredom and fatigue are the main causes. However, you can get the same effect by drinking a cup of coffee, because one tablet of NODOZ is equal to about one cup of coffee in caffeine content. It is not a good idea to take these products regularly because they cause the heart rate to speed up and may even affect blood circulation. Taking ten tablets or more a day could cause you to become physically dependent on them. However, taken only occasionally, they should not cause problems. If you suffer from heart problems or circulatory diseases, be sure to check with your doctor before taking any stimulant product.

When on trips many people will take these products when they start to feel tired while driving. It might be best to pull off the road, get out of the car, and stretch your muscles; this helps increase circulation throughout the body. And perhaps instead of taking a tablet, you might be better off relaxing and drinking a cup of coffee. You will feel rested and ready to continue your trip safely.

By the way, if you are driving on a long trip and notice your legs falling asleep, when you reach an area of highway where you can coast, let your foot off the accelerator and stretch it as far as you can; then wiggle your toes and shake your foot. This helps improve circulation and prevents areas of your body from falling asleep.

39

SUMMER AILMENTS

Everyone enjoys being outdoors—enjoying nature, playing sports, and going on picnics in the summertime. But you can develop HEAT EXHAUSTION or possibly HEAT STROKE, which may be life-threatening. It is important to know the difference between the two: With heat exhaustion the victim usually develop CRAMPS in the muscles, NAUSEA, and even VOMITING. The skin becomes PALE and CLAMMY, and he may black out. The best first aid is to get the person to a cool area and sponge down the skin with a cold, wet cloth. Once they regain consciousness, give them fluids to drink.

With heat stroke, on the other hand, mattters are much more serious. The person suffering from heat stroke FAINTS and the skin appears RED and fiery HOT. If you notice these symptoms, get the person into the shade, and try to lower the body temperature with either cold water or ice. Call for immediate help, or try to get the person to an emergency room.

The best thing to do during hot weather is to keep as cool as possible. Wear loose-fitting clothing in light colors rather than dark ones, because dark colors absorb more heat. If you perspire a lot, you may want to try taking a salt tablet to replenish the salt your body is losing. However, be careful when taking these tablets; they can cause IRRITATION to the stomach, leading to NAUSEA and VOMITING. Buffered salt tablets are available and are not so irritating to the stomach.

When perspiration evaporates, the body cools down. But perspiration has SALT in it, and if we lose too much salt, we become ill. If you must be in the heat, especially if you have a job where you are outside exercising or doing strenuous work, it might be a good idea to liberally salt the food you eat (unless your doctor has put you on a salt-free diet). Always drink lots of liquids, especially products such as GATORADE; they contain salts dissolved in the liquid to replace those your body is losing. If you don't have GATOR-ADE handy, try dissolving a teaspoonful of salt in a quart of lemonade or KOOL-AID and carry that with you. If you are affected by the heat, it would be a good idea to stay indoors or in the shade on very humid days, when there is a lot of moisture in the air and sweat cannot evaporate fast enough to cool the body properly. If you take the necessary precautions you can prevent serious effects of heat.

POISON IVY

No one is immune to poison ivy. Some people say that they can rub it all over them and they do not develop a rash. That might be true for a while. But as your body chemistry changes, so could its ability to resist effects of poison ivy. (When I was in college, I wanted to show everybody that I was immune to poison ivy, so I rubbed it all over my arms. Prior to that time I had touched the plant and never developed anything. However, this time I was covered with an angry rash and felt miserable for a few weeks.) Usually if you have a poison ivy rash, you have come into direct contact with the plant. But you can come into contact with it indirectly. For example, if your dog or cat runs into some bushes and the substance on the leaves of the plant gets on your pet's fur, when you pet old Rover you get poison ivy rash. Say a neighbor burns some weeds to get rid of them. The poison from the plant can be carried in the smoke and, you guessed it, if the smoke comes into contact with your skin, you develop a poison ivy reaction.

How do you know if you have a poison ivy rash? If you have been in the woods or some other place where there are weeds, and if the next day you develop ITCHING, SWELLING, and a streaky rash on the skin, you are doubtless the proud owner of a poison ivy reaction.

Poison ivy poisoning usually runs its course in about ten to fourteen days, and there is really very little one can do to stop it. However you can treat the symptoms, usually severe itching and a rash accompanied by little blisters that ooze a liquid when you scratch them. Years ago it was thought that the liquid caused the rash to spread. Let's set the record straight right now: The liquid that flows from the rash does not spread poison ivy rash on your own skin, much less somebody else's. It is the poisonous substance from the plant that causes the rash. If you scratch yourself and get that substance under your fingernails, everything you touch will cause an outbreak of the rash. If you come home from being outdoors and think you might have brushed against the plant, wash your clothing right away. Otherwise, every time you put on that favorite pair of jeans you will get poison ivy. If you have been all day in the woods and get home late, do not just take off your clothes and go to bed without a shower. If you have the substance on your skin it will rub off on the sheets, and every time you climb into bed you could cause a new outbreak of poison ivy reaction.

There are many products available to treat the poisoning. Some of them are intended to help dry up rash. IVY DRY contains TANNIC ACID, which helps stop the oozing of the blisters. Other products like CALADRYL, RHULIHIST, or ZIRADRYL have antihistamines in them. Antihistamines do help stop itching, but it is doubtful that they do much good when applied topically because of the poor absorption through the skin. Some products contain deadening ingredients to numb the skin, but people should be careful when using these products. If the skin is broken, products containing BENZOCAINE could themselves cause allergic reactions.

Since we do know that antihistamines stop itching, take one tablet of a cold or allergy product around the house and see if you get relief. An old stand-by for your recovery period is CALAMINE lotion. It is cheap, simple, and when it dries on the skin it forms a protective coating to prevent scratching and possible skin infection, which can spread rapidly.

Another way of stopping the itching is to soak fifteen to twenty minutes in a tub of hot water. The hot water will produce a numbing effect on the skin. Pat dry afterwards; do not rub dry, or you will start the itching all over again. Alternately, apply cold compresses to the affected area. Several times a day, wrap gauze bandages around it, take about a pint of cool water, add one teaspoonful of vinegar, and pour the solution over the bandage for about fifteen minutes. Remove the bandage and apply calamine lotion over the entire area. Some people claim that if you break open a VITAMIN E capsule and apply the gel to the affected area, the skin heals a lot faster. But remember, no matter what method you try, a poison ivy condition usually runs its course in ten to fourteen days, the first five of which are usually the most uncomfortable.

If you are affected by poison ivy near the eyes or genitals, do not fool around with over-the-counter products. See your doctor instead. The swelling could prevent urination if it is near the genitals and impaired vision if it is near the eyes.

If you are extremely allergic to poison ivy, it would be wise to check with an allergist. He may be able to reduce your sensitivity to the plant by giving allergy injections. If you are going to be outdoors, taking a weekend camping trip or vacation, you may want to make sure your first-aid kit has something in it to give you relief.

INSECT REPELLENTS

What's a picnic in the park, or a romp in the woods, without insect bites? Thanks to modern science, we now have insect repellents with which to spray ourselves. The problem with these products is that people usually spray only their arms and legs and end up with ten mosquito bites on their heads. Obviously, it is not very safe to spray your face or head, but products like 6-12 and OFF are available in liquid form and towelettes which you can rub on areas of the face, head, and neck. Always avoid getting the repellent in your eyes or mouth. Some repellents are good to spray on your clothing if you are going to a wooded area with ticks and chiggers. In any case, make sure to apply the repellent to all the areas exposed to mosquitoes. If you use aerosols, always hold them at least six inches away from your body when you spray them. Be sure to read the information on the repellent thoroughly before you use it.

Another group of products are sprayed around you, not on you, to kill insects. Now these products are claimed to have been jungle-tested. Sounds great, doesn't it? But all you want is one to kill bugs in your backyard. The problem with these products is that once you spray them, the wind carries them off to another area, leaving you exposed to the aerial attacks of the dreaded mosquito. These products do kill mosquitoes, though. If you decide to use them, hold the can firmly in your hand at all times and every time you see a mosquito in the vicinity, fill the area with spray and hope that the spray stays in place long enough to kill the insects. If you use these sprays around your patio, be careful; some of them will kill your plants.

New products to repel mosquitoes are SKEETER GO AWAY and SKEETER TABS. These products differ from the rest because you take them orally. These products are expensive. However, they contain VITAMIN B-1, or THIA-MINE, which you can buy in the vitamin section of your drugstore at around one-third the price of the insect repellent tablets. Just look for a bottle of THIAMINE CHLORIDE or VITAMIN B-1 100 mg. tablets. Take one tablet every three to four hours while you are outdoors. They do help repel mosquitoes, though maybe not all of them. And if you are bitten, the vitamin helps heal the bite much more quickly. How does it work? You will notice that vitamin

B-1 has a rather strong odor. Since it is a water-soluble vitamin, your body gets rid of what it doesn't need by partial excretion through the pores of the skin. When mosquitoes detect this odor, they stay away. This vitamin is also safe for children to take.

No one really knows if this vitamin helps repel chiggers and ticks as well. But if you are going for a hike in a wooded area, take vitamin B-1 and also use one of the spray repellents around your pants cuffs, socks, and openings in outer clothing. Chiggers are insects that can cause unbearable aggravation, and in the worst possible places. They usually go to the tight-fitting clothing areas, such as the socks and belt line, because of the build-up of the blood supply. Chiggers actually eat their way into the skin, and the saliva they release causes severe ITCHING. The only way to take care of the problem is to kill the little beast itself. Some people believe that sprinkling sulfur powder on the clothing that fits tightly prevents chiggers bites. There are products on the market to treat chigger bites. They dry on the skin and eventually smother the bug. Clear fingernail polish also works well. First soak yourself in a tub of hot water to relieve the itching. Pat yourself dry and apply clear fingernail polish to each bite and let it dry.

TICKS

There is really no preventative measure for avoiding ticks. However, you might spray one of the insect repellents around the open areas of your clothing: pants cuffs, buttonholes, and other areas where the tick could get to the skin. Since ticks must be attached for several hours before they cause infection, check for them frequently if you are likely to be exposed to them. Ticks can be removed easily by first covering the tick for several minutes with PETROLEUM JELLY, fingernail polish, or ISOPROPYL ALCOHOL, and then by pulling slowly and steadily with tweezers or fingers protected with facial tissue.

An antiseptic solution should be applied to the bite site to prevent infection. If you touched the tick with your bare hands, wash them thoroughly with soap and water. Secretions from the tick could be infective.

BEE AND WASP STINGS

Bee and wasp stings are painful, to say the least. You also run a risk of severe allergic reaction to the sting. Obviously, there is no way to prevent a bee or wasp sting, but if you are stung, take the right steps to treat the bite. Products that contain an antihistamine may be applied to the bite to stop the allergic reaction, but there are a few things you can do if you do not have them available. First remove the stinger from the bite and, whatever you do, do not squeeze the stinger. If you do, you will be injecting yourself with more of the poison. Remove it by gently sliding it out with your fingernail. After the stinger has been removed, do one of two things. Apply ice to the bite; that will actually slow the poison's entry into your system. Or make a thick paste of baking soda and water and apply it directly to the bite. Leave it there for about 30 minutes; it neutralizes the poison. You may also take an oral antihistamine if you have one handy. If the reaction seems to continue to get worse, get to an emergency room fast. After the pain and reaction from the bite has stopped, apply one of the HYDROCORTISONE creams or lotions for three or four days. This will help stop the ITCHING that usually occurs during the healing period. Some people are highly ALLERGIC to bee and wasp stings, to the point that a single bite could put them into shock or even result in death. If that is the case for you or your family, carry an emergency bee- and wasp-sting kit with you. One such kit is called ANA KIT. This is a prescription item, but it contains all the emergency items you need in the event of a bee or wasp sting, such as a ready-to-use syringe containing EPINEPHRINE, a tourniquet, and antihistamine tablets, along with complete instructions on how to use the kit properly. If you carry this kit around with you, make sure the epinephrine is always fresh and ready to use; you can check it by observing the color. If it begins turning an amber or brown color, get a fresh supply. Epinephrine opens the bronchials so that you can breath more easily. Store your ANA KIT in a cool dark place to keep it fresh longer.

40

SUN

Every person whose aim is to have fun in the sun here and abroad has probably experienced a SUNBURN. The painful REDNESS, SWELLING, and TENDERNESS of the skin are the results of being exposed too long to the sun's ultraviolet rays. Long-term exposure, even without severe burning, causes skin to age prematurely, resulting in a loss of elasticity, thinning, wrinkling, and drying. Cumulative exposure from childhood to adulthood may cause pre-cancerous skin conditions, and skin cancer may ensue. When you buy a suntan lotion you will see products with pretty exotic names, like TROPICAL BLEND or HAWAIIAN TROPIC. These oils almost give you a tan from reading the labels. It is true that OILS will give you a very lusterous tan. However, the oil actually magnifies the sun's rays, causing the sun to penetrate the skin more deeply. This in turn could cause a pretty severe burn, especially if you are in the sun for the first time in the season, or if you have sensitive skin.

Some suntan products have a sunscreen added to prevent sunburn. Sunscreen is an especially good idea if you are going out for the first time, or if you have sensitive skin. But some sunscreening agents are better than others. One of the best sunscreens available is PARA-AMINOBENZOIC ACID, better known as PABA.

Of course since these products do block out some of the harmful burning rays of the sun, your suntanning will take a lot longer. If the tanning process takes longer, you will avoid the PEELING and ITCHING that goes with a sunburn. Some of the sunscreen products that contain PABA are PABAFILM and PRESUN. These products have alcoholic bases, which makes them easy to apply. Make sure you apply them evenly, which will in turn give you an even tan. These products wash off the skin easily, so if you perspire a lot, or go in swimming, be sure to reapply them if you continue to be out in the sun. Products containing PABA that are also in cream and lotion form, such as SUNDOWN, stay on the skin longer then the products with alcohol bases. Some people develop a rash when using a product containing PABA, because they are allergic to it. In that case, pick a different sunscreen, which your pharmacist can help you select. For areas, such as your nose, ears, and lips, that are especially sensitive, coat them with an ointment such as ZINC OXIDE, which will block out the sun completely.

After you have begun a tan using a sunscreen, you may change to a suntan lotion or oil, which will enrich your tan without burning. Some hotels offer a suntanning process that consists of four or five different lotions. You start with the first bottle for a couple of days, then use the other lotions in succession. By the time you get to the last bottle, you are supposed to have a luxurious tan. This method is fine if your vacation lasts three to four weeks. But you can cut down the time and expense by using a good sunscreening lotion first, then an oil after the tanning process begins. Even baby oil works at that point; the natural oil in your skin will also help promote a tan.

SUNBURN

Normally the healing process for sunburn takes two to three days. But those two or three days can be misery, especially if you are on vacation to enjoy yourself. Among the products available to relieve the pain of a sunburn are SOLARCAINE or RHULICAINE; these products contain an ingredient called BENZOCAINE which deadens the skin. They are available in creams, lotions, and sprays. Sprays are easier to use. After all, when you have a severe sunburn, you can hardly touch the skin, much less rub a lotion on it. Be careful when using these products, especially if you have blisters or broken skin; spraying them on broken skin can cause ALLERGIC REACTIONS or further IRRITATION to your skin. Another good treatment is to fill the bathtub with cool water, then submerge the sunburned area in the cool water for about thirty minutes. It will soothe the sunburn and relieve the pain temporarily, probably just as much as the anesthetic sprays. Also, you could take an oral pain reliever like ASPIRIN, which helps relieve INFLAMMATION, and so gives some relief for sunburn. If you cannot take aspirin, try one of the non-aspirin pain relievers, such as TYLENOL. You might also try a lotion with ALOE VERA, which has been shown to give relief from all types of burns.

A few additional things to keep in mind if you are going to be out in the sun: If you shower before going out, avoid using deodorant. It dries out the skin and washes away the skin's protective coating, making the skin more susceptible to the sun. Certain medications may cause the skin to become super-sensitive to the sun, resulting in more severe sunburn. Some drugs that cause this are the TETRACYCLINE antibiotics, certain tranquilizers, such as VALIUM and barbiturates, and THIAZIDE diuretics. The best advice pertaining to medications is to tell your pharmacist or doctor what drugs you are presently taking. If you are taking one that reacts with the sun, take the appropriate steps by using a sunscreen or avoid long exposure to the sun.

SUNGLASSES

The glare from the sun causes unnecessary squinting and EYE STRAIN, perhaps resulting in a HEADACHE. Obviously the best thing to do to prevent these problems is to wear a good pair of sunglasses. Of course, the best sunglasses are those obtained from an optical store. Such stores not only specialize in glasses of all kinds, but you can be assured of getting the most finely ground lenses available to suit your particular eyes. Unfortunately, you also pay a higher price for these glasses. This usually sends you into the drugstore to buy sunglasses off the bargain rack. The price will definitely meet the requirements of your pocketbook, but the glasses may not meet the requirements of your eyes. Often the sunglasses found on the bargain racks have actual flaws in the lenses. They may appear as scratches or bubbles in the lenses. These may cause unnecessary eye strain, which could result in a severe headache, or even NAUSEA and VOMITING.

There are other things to look for when you are buying sunglasses. Examine both lenses carefully; make sure they are the same color and shade. Hold them away from your face and look at a straight line somewhere through each lens. You can use a line in the ceiling of the store or a corner of the building. Make sure that the line is perfectly straight. If the lens causes the straight line to appear wavy, this may also cause unnecessary eye strain and the annoying problems that go along with it.

Selecting the right color lens is sometimes just as important as making sure that the lenses have no flaws. The best way to select the color of the lenses is to know what you want them to do for you. Dark gray lenses are most effective at blocking out the sun. They also give a true lifelike color to the objects you look at. Another effective color for blocking out the sun is a brown lens. Brown lenses appear to brighten up the objects you look at. This could be important to a fisherman, for example. The lens not only blocks out the sun, but you are able to see the cork better when the big ones are biting. Yellow lenses do not do a thing to block out the sun's rays, but they brighten everything. That is why one often see skiers wearing them. They give a definite outline to the objects you see. As far as rose-colored lenses go, life does not look rosier through these lenses. They are mainly used for cosmetic purposes along with green and blue lenses. However, rose-colored lenses do help to some degree to reduce the glare of fluorescent lights. So if you work in an office, where the fluorescent lights cause a glare on your work, maybe even resulting in periodic headaches, you might want to try working with rose-colored lenses. People also seem to like photo-sensitive lenses, which darken as they are exposed to increased light. These are fine for some conditions, but if you are going to be on the beach or in the snow, where the sun is very bright, most photo-sensitive lenses do not get dark enough to block out the sun's rays effectively. No matter what color lenses you end up buying, make sure the lenses are free from flaws.

41

VACATION

Vacations are supposed to be a time for relaxation and enjoyment, but sometimes in their haste to get away from it all, people overlook certain aspects of travel that can prove hazardous to their health.

TRAVELLERS' DIARRHEA

This problem goes under many names such as "Montezuma's Revenge," "Runs," and "Dehli Belly." Whatever one calls it, it is a villain that terrorizes many travellers every year. The most common cause is bacteria in the water, which produces a sudden onset of NAUSEA, CRAMPS, and DIARRHEA. Some experts say that not only the water but also environmental changes and unfamiliar foods and beverages can alter the intestinal flora, causing diarrhea.

Travellers' diarrhea generally disappears in two or three days, and one recommended treatment consists of rest, lots of fluids (especially for children), and simply letting it run its course. However, the use of KAOPECTATE and PEPTO-BISMOL is very effective in treating diarrhea, because they contain ingredients that act as a sponge in the intestine to absorb impurities. They also may be given to children. However, if you take the right precautions, you won't develop this problem.

You have heard the expression "Don't drink the water"; remember that this applies to ice cubes as well. Always boil water you are not sure about, and this includes bottled water if you are not sure of its source. You can also use water purification tablets, such as HALAZONE, and you outdoors people and campers can purify your water by placing five drops of TINCTURE OF IODINE from your first-aid kit in a quart of water and letting it stand for about fifteen minutes before using. Eat hot, thoroughly cooked meals if possible, and avoid fresh fruit and vegetables unless peeled and washed by trusted hands, namely your own. If you notice blood in the stool, check with a doctor. More rarely, some people may develop constipation while travelling because of sudden changes in their eating habits. This can usually be remedied by taking a stool softener like COLACE or DIALOSE or simply using MILK OF MAGNESIA.

MOTION SICKNESS

Many people get motion sickness while travelling by sea, air, or land. The main symptoms of motion sickness are NAUSEA and VOMITING. For people who suffer from motion sickness every time they travel, prevention is much easier than treatment after the symptoms have appeared. Some steps can be taken to avoid motion sickness. One is to sit in a position least likely to have exposure to ascending motion. For example, if you often develop motion sickness when travelling by airplane, try sitting in a seat between the wings of the plane. It may spoil your view, but how much can you see anyway when you are staring into a barf bag? Sitting in a semi-reclined position will also help. Reading or unusual visual stimulation should be avoided.

People who usually develop motion sickness should avoid eating or drinking too much before leaving on a trip. While on the trip, only fluids and simple foods should be consumed.

There are products available for motion sickness, such as BONINE, DRAMAMINE, EMETROL, and MAREZINE. These antinauseants should be taken 30 minutes to an hour before the trip. They do work well at preventing motion sickness, and some are available in liquid form for children. But since they are chemically related to antihistamines, they sometimes cause excessive DROWSINESS and SLEEPINESS. So if you decide to take one of these products, let someone else do the driving.

STORING MEDICINE

People who take medicines routinely for various problems, such as high blood pressure, diabetes, etc., must be sure to pack their medicines along with all the other items they take on vacation. Be sure to keep your medicine in its original prescription bottle with the label on it. People sometimes want to put their pills in smaller containers to carry them. If you are going to do this, ask your pharmacist to give you a smaller bottle with a prescription label on it. You never know when an emergency might happen. If you need treatment, a doctor can easily look at your prescription bottle to get the name of the medicines you are taking and know what treatment would be best for you.

Another good reason to keep your medicines in their original bottles with the label on them is in the event that you are stopped by the local authorities. If they find an unmarked bottle of medicine, it could cause some unnecessary harassment. When you are travelling, avoid putting your medicines into a suitcase and throwing them in the trunk of the car. Excessive heat causes some medicines to deteriorate. If you are going to carry medicines with you and you are travelling in a car, keep the medicine in the glove compartment. As an added safety precaution, keep the glove compartment locked.

If you travel by airplane, bus, or train, it is a good idea not to pack your medicine in a suitcase that will be placed in the luggage compartment, but to keep it in a case that you can carry with you. Luggage sometimes gets lost, but if you carry an overnight case, you won't be without your medicine while the luggage is located.

Some people develop congestion in the ears due to changes in pressure when travelling by airplane. Usually yawning or chewing gum opens them up. But some people have a difficult time keeping them open. You might want to try an inhaler, such as **BENZEDREX INHALER,** that is recommended for use in air travel. It contains a decongestant to keep the sinuses open, which helps to keep the ears open as well. If that doesn't help, try taking a decongestant tablet such as **SUDAFED** before your trip.

As a precaution against losing your medicine or leaving it sitting at home, have your doctor write you a new prescription for all the medicines you take before you leave on your trip. Keep those written prescriptions in your wallet, or some other safe place, so that you can have them filled at a nearby pharmacy should you need them.

DIABETICS sometimes have problems with medicine while travelling, especially if they have to inject themselves with **INSULIN.** Although insulin should be refrigerated, you may keep it in your car; it will stay fresh as long as you have an air conditioner that keeps the inside of the car cool and close to normal room temperature. If you do not have an air conditioner, fill a small plastic bag with ice. Then put your insulin in another plastic bag and place that in the bag of ice. Close up the bag tightly to prevent it from leaking in the car. As long as you can keep replenishing your ice supply, you will keep your insulin cool and ready for use.

No matter what kind of medicine you take, after you arrive at your destination, check into a hotel, and unpack your suitcase, you might want to keep your medicine in one of the empty suitcases, locked up. Do not set your medicine in the bathroom or on the night stand in your room; you may find it missing.

42
VITAMINS

Americans are popping more pills than ever before, and some of those pills are being popped in the name of good health. I am talking about vitamins. Many people feel that they need vitamins nowadays because of the hectic lives they lead and the fact that they often do not eat well. It is not wrong to take vitamins; after all, they are essential to life itself. However, some health food advocates tell you that vitamins are the answer to many problems. Americans must believe it, because they spend over $400 million dollars a year on vitamin products.

Actually vitamins are useful to some individuals, such as growing children, the elderly who often cannot properly absorb certain vitamins from the foods they eat, or the person recuperating from an illness. However, in many cases the average American diet does not need additional vitamin supplements. If we are as vitamin-deficient as some people claim, why are vitamin deficiency illnesses not reported? Marketing practices have confused the issue further with the words "organic" or "natural."

Is there a difference in these products? Yes: The natural is more expensive than the synthetic. The reason the natural or organic product is more expensive is that it is extracted from foods without the use of chemicals or additives, and the foods that they are extracted from are grown without the use of agricultural chemicals. But there is no evidence that organically grown food is more nutritious than foods grown using chemical fertilizers, although questions have been raised about the safety of ingesting chemicals such as fertilizers, pesticides, and preservatives.

It has also been found that "natural" vitamins frequently are supplemented by the synthetic vitamin. For example, the amount of ASCORBIC ACID extracted from rose hips is relatively small, and sometimes synthetic VITAMIN C is added to bring it up to the strength it is supposed to be. This addition is not shown on the label, and such products always cost a lot more than the synthetic and equally effective vitamin.

Once again I am not saying that it is wrong to take vitamins. Take the multiple vitamin and mineral combination to get enough vitamins and minerals, but not too much of any one vitamin. Problems can develop if you start taking individual vitamins; some are fat-soluble, which means that what your body does not use it stores in the fat cells. These vitamins can reach a very high level and produce side effects, some of them serious. Certainly vitamins are needed to help each other work properly. Vitamin A, for instance, helps the body use CALCIUM, and vitamin C helps us use IRON more effectively.

Always be sure that the vitamins you buy are fresh. Check the package for an expiration date.

When giving vitamins to children, always refer to them as medicine and not candy. Chewable vitamins are frequently given to children. Nowadays there are a wide variety of brands to choose from: FLINTSTONES, BUGS BUNNY, STRAWBERRY SHORTCAKE, and MONSTER, to name a few. They are pleasant-tasting and come in the shapes of various cartoon or other characters. Since vitamins are important to growing children, for strong bones and teeth, it would not hurt to give them one of these chewable vitamins each day, especially if they do not always eat properly. However, if children associate the vitamins with candy, someday when you are out of the room they may eat the contents of an entire bottle, thinking it is nothing more than candy. And there can be serious side effects from too much of certain vitamins, such as VITAMINS **A, D, E,** and **K.**

If you are watching your pennies, and who isn't nowadays, check different brands as well as the amount of the vitamin in each tablet. Then buy one that has a low cost per unit of vitamin. Many stores have their own brands, which will save you money.

FAT-SOLUBLE VITAMINS

These are VITAMINS **A, D,** and E. Severe deficiencies of any of these vitamins may result in conditions as serious as blindness or bone deformity, and excessive doses may be harmful. Do not exceed the recommended dosage, which is usually based on the U.S. Recommended Daily Allowance (RDA).

VITAMIN A

This vitamin is needed to prevent night blindness and the drying of the membrane at the corner of the eye. A deficiency of VITAMIN A can also cause dryness of the skin or other areas of the body. Pregnant women must have an adequate supply of vitamin A. Good natural sources of vitamin A are kidney, milk products, eggs, fish liver oil, and palm oil. Skim milk is not a good source of vitamin A because the milk fat, where the vitamin is stored, has been removed. As a matter of fact, severe vitamin A deficiency was reported in Brazil because their sole diet was skim milk. So if you drink skim milk, you had better take additional vitamin A. Some of the signs and symptoms of vitamin A deficiency related to the eye are DRYING, WRINKLING, and HAZING of the cornea. These problems become evident more rapidly in children than in adults. Most people can take between

25,000 and 50,000 units of vitamin A daily without any problem. Side effects have resulted when people take ten to twenty times this dosage, including FATIGUE, NAUSEA, JOINT PAIN, throbbing HEADACHES, BRITTLE NAILS, and ROUGH SCALY SKIN. If you take vitamin A and any of these signs develop, stop taking it, and check with your doctor.

VITAMIN D

The "sunshine vitamin" is needed to help the body absorb and use calcium, which is needed for strong bones and teeth, from the small intestine. Inadequate vitamin D results in a condition known as "RICKETS." Sometimes vitamin D deficiencies are caused by KIDNEY DISEASE. Natural sources of vitamin D are fish liver oils, sunlight, and yeast. Some foods are artificially fortified with vitamin D, including milk and cereals. The signs of vitamin D deficiency disease are calcium problems, specifically problems in bone formation, such as RICKETS, which is evident as soft bones and deformed joints.

Since this vitamin can be stored in the body, excessive amounts produce side effects such as LOSS OF APPETITE, NAUSEA, WEAKNESS, WEIGHT LOSS, FREQUENT URINATION, and high levels of calcium in the blood, which could cause the formation of kidney stones. Doctors will sometimes prescribe liquid vitamin D for infants. If you use this product, be sure to measure the amount you give the child very carefully.

VITAMIN E

This is probably the most controversial of all the vitamins, especially in the last few years; various claims have been made for its use, such as to increase your sex drive or grow hair. We do know at least that VITAMIN E is essential to life. Vitamin E seems necessary in preventing problems involving the muscles, nerves, and the blood vessels.

One of the main sources of vitamin E is soybean, and

since the American diet now includes more soybean products, it is almost impossible to have a deficiency of vitamin E. Other sources of vitamin E are vegetable oils, particularly safflower oil, nuts, and cereals. Large doses of vitamin E have not been shown to produce significant side effects. However, since it is stored up in our bodies, it is not a good idea to take over 800 units per day over a long period of time. If you should notice symptoms such as NAUSEA and HEADACHES, check with your doctor. Patients were given daily doses of 400 to 3200 units of vitamin E and some cases reported improvement. However, more studies are needed, particularly of its effects on ANGINA and FIBROCYSTIC DISEASE, which is a painful condition of the breast. Attempting to self-treat a potentially serious symptom such as CHEST PAIN with vitamin E only delays proper medical treatment. Taking vitamin E along with IRON products can be counterproductive, since iron causes the body to eliminate vitamin E more rapidly.

WATER-SOLUBLE VITAMINS

The water-soluble vitamins are ASCORBIC ACID, THIAMINE HYDROCHLORIDE, RIBOFLAVIN, NIACIN, PYRIDOXINE HYDROCHLORIDE, CYANOCOBALAMINE, FOLIC ACID, PANTOTHENIC ACID, BIOTIN, RIBOFLAVINOIDS, CHOLINE, and INOSITOL. Water-soluble means that what our body does not use is excreted. Such vitamins are the reason that our urine turns bright yellow after we take a multiple vitamin. Our system is flushing the excess out.

ASCORBIC ACID (VITAMIN C)

Ascorbic acid has become a sort of super folk-hero vitamin, said to aid, for instance, in the prevention of colds. According to a leading medical journal, a study was conducted at West Point in which one group of cadets were given PLACEBOS (sugar pills), the other group, vitamin C. The results of the study showed that the group that took vitamin C had more colds than the other group. However, another recent study showed that vitamin C could be useful in preventing BACTERIAL INFECTIONS, so that colds due to bacteria might be prevented by vitamin C.

Actually, humans must consume ascorbic acid daily because it is not produced by our bodies. People who smoke should take additional vitamin C, because smokers show a decreased level of vitamin C. Ascorbic acid is responsible for healthy teeth and gums. It is also responsible for wound healing. If we are deficient in vitamin C, our wounds heal slowly or old ones reopen, and the gums may become swollen and bleed easily. If not treated, this could result in death. Large doses of vitamin C during pregnancy could cause the child to be born with REBOUND SCURVY. Since vitamin C is a water-soluble vitamin, it enters the systems of both mother and child, resulting in the infant requiring higher doses of vitamin C than normal after birth. If normal doses are then given, the infant may develop the vitamin C deficiency disease called SCURVY.

The most common early symptom of vitamin C deficiency is ROUGH SKIN, which is experienced most often in the winter when fresh fruits and vegetables are not plentiful. A more serious symptom is EASY BRUISING. The recommended daily allowance of vitamin C is 50 mg., though some people take 500 mg. Though such a dosage probably won't cause any harm, it is very doubtful that it will do any good. However, larger doses of vitamin C may cause DIARRHEA and, since it acidifies the urine, the formation of KIDNEY STONES.

DIABETICS should be careful when taking vitamin C. They must test their urine periodically to make sure that their diabetes is under control. Vitamin C can alter these readings. Vitamin C should be avoided when taking blood-thinning drugs like COUMADIN and DICUMAROL. Vitamin C also helps our bodies use IRON properly.

VITAMIN B-1 (THIAMINE)

THIAMINE is responsible for breaking down fats and carbohydrates into energy. This in turn keeps the vital organs, such as the heart, muscles, and nervous systems, functioning properly. A good source of vitamin B-1 is the hull of rice grains. Other good sources are pork, beef, fresh peas, and beans. Thiamine deficiencies occur in ALCOHOLICS and other people who have been VOMITING for a long period of time. Thiamine's toxicity is relatively mild because it is a water-soluble vitamin, and our body gets rid of what it does not need in the urine. Thiamine is mainly used to supplement the diets of people who have poor dietary habits due to alcoholism.

VITAMIN B COMPLEX

Many vitamin products sold today consist of a combination of all the B vitamins, such as THIAMINE, RIBOFLAVIN, NIACIN, PYRIDOXINE, and CYANOCOBALAMINE.

RIBOFLAVIN is responsible for cellular growth. If you become deficient in riboflavin, you may develop a crack in the corner of the mouth or the lip. Taking riboflavin or the B-complex for a couple of days will usually clear it up.

NIACIN is available either as niacin (NICOTINIC ACID) or as NIACINAMIDE. Both work the same way, but niacin causes flushing of the skin and niacinamide doesn't. Foods rich in niacin are beef, cow's milk, and whole eggs. Deficiencies of niacin are evident as a thickening of the skin on the face, which may look like a severe burn. Niacin should not be taken by people suffering from ULCERS or other chronic stomach problems. Sometimes niacin can trigger ASTHMA ATTACKS.

PYRIDOXINE is essential in nutrition and is especially important in infants and children, as well as in pregnant or lactating women. The symptoms of pyridoxine deficiency are CONVULSIONS—in which a person becomes unconscious, with uncontrollable tremors or shaking—and IRRITABILITY.

Foods rich in pyridoxine are meats, cereals, lentils, nuts, and some fruits and vegetables, such as bananas, avocados, and potatoes. Cooking destroys some of the vitamin, and artificial infant formulas are required to contain pyridoxine. Several drugs affect pyridoxine's use in the body, including ISONIAZID and CYCLOSERINE (SEROMYCIN) (antitubercular drugs), as well as HYDRALAZINE for high blood pressure. Women taking ESTROGEN in birth control pills will also get rid of too much pyridoxine and may want to supplement their diet. Pyridoxine may block the effects of a prescription drug known as LEVODOPA, used for PARKINSON'S DISEASE. In that case, pyridoxine should be avoided as much as possible.

CYANOCOBALAMINE is necessary for many cellular activities, and it also plays a big role in breaking down fats and carbohydrates for energy. It is present in animal protein and micro-organisms. Vegetarians may need to supplement their diets with additional cyanocobalamine, since it is important in cell production. If you are deficient in this vitamin, you develop STOMACH PROBLEMS, INFLAMMATION of the tongue, SORE MOUTH, and DIARRHEA. Some prescription drugs such as NEOMYCIN and COLCHICINE may cause cyanocobalamine not to be absorbed properly.

Rather than using any of the B vitamins individually, you might be better off with the B complex, because it is often difficult to pinpoint the exact B vitamin that you are lacking. Since B works in combination, with the B complex you should be getting adequate protection.

MINERALS

Many vitamin preparations are available with minerals, such as UNICAP-M, THERAGRAN-M, or the store brand multivitamins with minerals. As a matter of fact, if you are going to supplement your diet with a multiple vitamin, why not get one with minerals? That way you are getting everything from A to Z, and they do not cost much more. Some of the most common minerals found in vitamin products are:

IRON

IRON DEFICIENCY ANEMIA is a widespread problem. Although it has caused few deaths, it contributes to poor health and sub-optimal performance in many people. Iron deficiency anemia may result from inadequate diet, inability to absorb iron properly, pregnancy and lactation, or blood loss. Only about ten percent of the iron in food or iron supplements is absorbed into our system. Usually women need supplemental iron more than men, especially if they have heavy menstrual periods. Early symptoms of iron deficiency are FATIGUE and WEAKNESS. (These symptoms could also be related to other illnesses.) Other symptoms of anemia are DIFFICULTY IN BREATHING, PALE COLOR, COLDNESS, and NUMBNESS of the extremities.

Before buying an iron preparation, it might be a good idea to check with your doctor or pharmacist first. If iron products are suggested, there are many to choose from. How do you know which one to use? You might take a multivitamin with iron. Or you might use an iron supplement by itself. If you decide to use an iron supplement, look at the ingredients to know what to expect from the product you are about to buy.

FERROUS SULFATE is found in many iron preparations; however, this source tends to irritate the stomach, producing NAUSEA and STOMACH PAIN. FERROUS FUMARATE as well as FERROUS GLUCONATE, also found in some iron preparations, are a little less irritating to the stomach.

Some iron products are available in combination with VITAMIN C, which helps the body use iron more effectively. No matter what iron preparation you choose, one common side effect is CONSTIPATION. You can remedy this by taking a stool softener periodically. Another thing you might notice when taking iron is that the stool becomes BLACK and TARRY. This is the result of the unabsorbed iron. If you take iron and sometimes find that it causes NAUSEA, VOMITING, or DIARRHEA, it might help to take it with food, either while you are eating or immediately after you finish your meal. If after taking it for one month, there is no improvement, check with your doctor. You should notice some relief of your anemia symptoms in 30 days. By the same token, if you are just starting to take an iron product, only buy a month's supply, so that if it does not work for you, you won't be wasting your money.

Iron may react with certain prescription drugs, such as TETRACYCLINE, causing it not to be absorbed properly. It is also recommended that you avoid taking iron if you are taking ALLOPURINOL (ZYLOPRIM).

CALCIUM

Calcium is the main component of teeth and bones, and it also plays a major role in clotting the blood. Deficiencies of this mineral can cause BRITTLE BONES or SOFT TEETH. Calcium is available without a prescription in the form of CALCIUM CARBONATE, CALCIUM GLUCONATE, and CALCIUM LACTATE. However, calcium should only be taken by itself under the orders of your doctor, because it may be toxic and if high levels build up in the urine, could cause the formation of KIDNEY STONES.

TRACE ELEMENTS (ZINC AND COPPER)

Other minerals are needed by the body only in small quantities, but they are essential. ZINC, for instance, is necessary for the healing of wounds. Inadequate zinc consumption may cause a blunting of the senses of taste and smell, and POOR APPETITE and POOR GROWTH may occur in children with low zinc intake. COPPER helps maintain adequate blood-cell production.

MEGAVITAMINS

Although MEGAVITAMIN therapy has been used with success in certain patient populations, there is no evidence to indicate that large doses of vitamins ensure good health. Indeed, some serious side effects have been reported. One sees many new products, such as GINSENG, KELP, LECITHIN, etc., in the vitamin sections of drugstores. However, the nutrients in these products have not been proven medically, and chances are that you are getting more than enough of the ingredients in these products in your normal diet. Since some of these products cause problems for people suffering from DIABETES or HIGH BLOOD PRESSURE, do not be swayed to use them without proper medical advice. Most of the people pushing these products are more interested in your money than your health.

If you are interested in more than this basic information, talk to your doctor or to the local hospital dietician.

I truly believe that nutrition is important for good health and that a lot more research should be done in this area. But remember that fad diets are no substitute for sound medical care; let your doctor be the judge.

APPENDIX: DRUG ABUSE

Drug abuse is a problem growing to epidemic proportions. It is something to which no one is immune; it is a problem facing many teenagers and a serious concern of their parents as well. The following information was put together by the National Council on Drug Abuse and, we hope, will help you and your children better understand drugs and their uses and abuses.

Drugs are all around us. Some, like tobacco, alcohol, and coffee, are generally accepted and are even looked upon by many as useful substances. These drugs are in use daily, and some adults abuse them with little thought of the influence such abuse may have on younger people.

We use a wide variety of legal prescription and nonprescription drugs, including stimulants (like AMPHETAMINES, CAFFEINE, NICOTINE) and depressants (like SLEEPING PILLS, TRANQUILIZERS, ALCOHOL), as well as numerous over-the-counter drugs, to relieve nearly every kind of human ailment, real or imagined. When used properly, most of these drugs are helpful. Unfortunately, an increasing number of people misuse these drugs by taking them for the wrong reason, or too frequently, or in combinations that sometimes create highly dangerous drug interactions.

Then there are drugs with marginal social acceptance, substances like MARIJUANA and HASHISH, that are still illegal, but are used by a growing number of Americans. The long-term effects of these drugs are being studied, but we know that they are by no means harmless. As with all drugs, there is always the danger of abuse, which can lead to serious physical, emotional, and mental side effects. Until more is known, the wisest course is to avoid drugs of this sort. One unfortunate result of their use has been the conflict between the young and their elders. Those who use these drugs may become secretive and isolated; they often feel that they must lie to cover their actions, and sometimes turn to petty crimes to gain money to buy the drugs illegally.

Finally there are drugs that are both clearly dangerous and illegal like HEROIN, LSD, and PCP, and that when taken alone or together with other substances may have severe effects upon the user. All drugs, legal and illegal, prescription and over-the-counter, are available with varying ease to children as well as to adults, poor and rich. More detailed information of the effects of these and other commonly used drugs will be given later.

The widespread availability of these substances is itself a problem, but the wrong reaction will only worsen that problem. You may not be able to stop the flow of drugs, but you can help to keep it from involving people you care about. You can do this because, by understanding the problem and the solution, you can attack its very root.

The reasons that people abuse drugs are as different and varied as the people themselves, but in general people seem to take drugs to change the way they feel. They may want to feel better or to feel happy. They may want to escape from pain, stress, or frustration. They may want to forget or to remember, to be accepted or to be sociable. Sometimes people take drugs to escape boredom, or just to satisfy their curiosity. At certain times during a young person's life, peer pressure can be a very strong reason to use drugs. People often feel better about themselves when they use drugs or alcohol, but the effects don't last. Drugs never solve problems, they only postpone them. In the long run, people who misuse or abuse drugs in the hope of solving one problem run the risk of getting trapped in a spiral of increasing drug use that creates new problems and makes old problems worse.

Prevention should be a positive idea, not a negative one. Prevention is building a resistance to abusing drugs before it begins. Prevention includes a wide range of efforts to help people develop skills and talents, to help them become confident and have a sense of their own worth, to help them learn to make wise decisions about their bodies and lives. If people are confident and generally feel good about themselves, they will be less likely to abuse drugs. Stated another way, prevention means replacing the negative feelings about oneself with strong positive attitudes and values. Here are some of the things we all need to help us avoid the temptation to abuse drugs.

- Love, affection, and attention from those we care about.
- Consistent and fair discipline and encouragement.
- Opportunities to express our feelings and thoughts.
- Opportunities for successful and exciting experiences at home, in school, at work, and in the community.
- Tolerance for mistakes.
- Models of strong and thoughtful people to look up to.
- Accurate information about the problems of society today: sexuality, drugs, crime, and other issues that threaten us or make us fearful.

While this may sound obvious, studies of serious drug abusers show that they have failed to receive the simple kinds of support described above.

Prevention may be as easy as providing alternative outlets and interesting activities, such as sports, crafts, music, and recreation, to name just a few. It may mean improving relationships between adults and young people through community discussion groups, counselling centers, or other activities involving both groups. Community drug abuse prevention means getting people (parents, young people, adults who work with young people, all people young or old) involved in mutually satisfying and rewarding activities. The answer depends on who you are. Different people can do different things to help prevent drug abuse.

Because the best time to prevent drug abuse is between the ages of eight and twenty, families are very important. Prevention can be as easy as helping your children find satisfying alternatives to drugs. If you don't already know what your children like to do best, take the time to find out. Take the time to do what they enjoy. Too often other things seem more important. To prevent drug abuse, there is nothing more important then spending time with your children. In its simplest form, prevention is being there when you are needed. It is providing love and guidance for the children. It is helping them learn about the world with the support and supervision of people who care. It is establishing limits to protect them from situations they aren't ready to handle. It is trying to maintain a balance in their lives.

In studies comparing adolescent users and non-users of drugs, we have learned that what often separates the two groups are human qualities that develop over many years and have a lot to do with the relationships and trust among members of a family. Close, caring families may be practicing prevention without being aware of it.

Most young people who don't use drugs report that their parents treat them with respect, that their parents listen to them, and that their families help them solve problems. Families who listen to each other and share their feelings are the most important factor in preventing drug abuse.

Among their peers, young people are constantly subjected to group pressure, pressure to fit in, to be accepted. This pressure can either encourage or discourage drug use and abuse. For young people prevention may mean being there when a friend needs help. Problems that seem too big for one person alone can usually be solved if others help.

Growing up is never easy, and sometimes drugs seem like the best way to get away from problems. But those problems will still be waiting when the high is over, often accompanied by new ones caused by drug abuse. To prevent these new problems from developing, young people must help each other over the rough spots that can lead to drugs, and everyone must have a basic understanding of drugs and their effects. The following information will help you better understand.

A drug is any chemical substance that brings about physical, emotional, or mental changes in people. Alcohol, tobacco, and even caffeine in coffee, tea, cocoa, and cola drinks are drugs. Other less widely used drugs include **THC** in MARIJUANA and HASHISH, AMPHETAMINES, BAR-BITURATES, TRANQUILIZERS, NARCOTICS, COCAINE, PHENCYCLIDINE **(PCP),** volatile chemicals, GLUE and other inhalants, and **LSD.**

Drug abuse is the use of a chemical substance, legal or illegal, which causes physical, mental, emotional, or social harm to a person or to people close to him or her.

There are different kinds of drug users. Experimental users may try various drugs once or twice out of curiosity about their effects. Recreational users use drugs regularly to achieve or maintain a desired state, but attempt to continue normal activity. Dependent users cannot relate to anything but drug-seeking and drug-taking. They experience mental or physical discomfort when they need drugs and will do anything to obtain them. All drugs can be harmful. The effect of any drug depends on a lot of things, including how much is taken, how often, the way it is taken (smoking, taking pills, etc.), whether other drugs are taken at the same time, the user's personality, and the setting, the place, and the other people.

Multiple drug use is very common and very dangerous. People who use one kind of drug are more likely to use other kinds of drugs too, either one after another or at the same time. Greater risks exist when a combination of drugs or a mixture of pills is taken. A common example of multiple drug use is the use of alcohol and sleeping pills together, which can lead to RESPIRATORY FAILURE and COMA or DEATH.

Drug use is often hard to detect, especially in the early stages. Of course, many drugs have some effect in common or have different effects at different times. Dependence exists when people like drugs or feel they need drugs so much that they cannot do without them. Only a few kinds of drugs, like NARCOTICS, can cause physical dependence or ADDICTION. But almost any drug, when used regularly or misused, can make a person think they need the drug—that is, can make a person psychologically dependent. Let's take a quick look at three very common drugs, sometimes called the "gateway drugs," because they are the ones most of us come into contact with first.

TOBACCO

NICOTINE, the active ingredient in tobacco, acts as a stimulant to the heart and nervous system. When a cigarette smoker inhales tobacco smoke into the lungs, the heart beats faster and blood pressure rises. Smoking is the nation's most widespread, costly, and physically dangerous addiction. Addiction to nicotine exists in one-third of our population. Long-term use leads to physical illnesses like LUNG and HEART DISEASE and CANCER.

ALCOHOL

ETHYL ALCOHOL is the active ingredient in wine, beer, and liquors. In small doses, it has a calming effect, like all depressants. An occasional drink is usually not harmful and may in fact have some good effects. However, if even a few drinks are taken rapidly, the small blood vessels can be blocked and some tissues and cells can be deprived of needed oxygen. Taken in larger quantities over long periods of time, alcohol damages the liver, brain, and heart. Repeated use of alcohol can cause PERMANENT BRAIN DAMAGE and impaired memory, judgment, and learning.

Alcoholism has long been recognized as a major problem in our country. The National Clearinghouse on Alcohol Information has free information about the misuse and abuse of alcohol for anyone who asks for it. Write to

National Clearinghouse on Alcohol Information
Box 2345
Rockville, Maryland 20852

MARIJUANA AND HASHISH

The use of MARIJUANA and HASHISH has increased greatly among Americans during the last decade. There is still a great deal not known about this drug, but scientists are learning more about its effects. Marijuana (called "pot," "grass," "weed"), HASHISH, and HASHISH OIL come from a plant named *Cannabis sativa*. The dried, chopped leaves are called marijuana. The dark brown resin from the tops of the plant is hashish. Hash oil is distilled from hashish.

All parts of the cannabis plant derive their effects primarily from a drug called DELTA-9-TETRA-HYDRO-CANNABINOL, THC for short. Smoking or eating THC brings most of the high. Even though it is an illegal drug, marijuana use generally continues to increase among young and not-so-young people. It has been established that about 30 million Americans have tried marijuana. There is still much to be learned about the long-range effects of marijuana. There is good evidence, however, that marijuana can be harmful. On the immediate level, tests have shown that marijuana impairs the ability to drive or perform other complex tasks. Long-term use is still being studied. Among the major areas of study are

- Harm to the body's natural defense system.
- Basic alterations in cell metabolism.
- Possible reduction in the male hormone testosterone and in growth hormone levels.
- Reduction of motivation and constructive energy.

There is reason enough to be concerned about marijuana use in all age groups, but young persons especially are still developing their personalities and bodies and might be more sensitive to the long-range effects.

THE STIMULANTS

Stimulants are the "uppers" that excite the nervous system. They relieve DROWSINESS and disguise the effects of FATIGUE and EXHAUSTION. The stronger stimulants sometimes produce a temporary EUPHORIA (high mood). Using stimulants regularly makes some people IRRITABLE and OVERACTIVE. People who use stimulants over a long period of time and then stop can go through a WITHDRAWAL and may feel ANXIOUS, DEPRESSED, or get HEADACHES or other symptoms.

CAFFEINE

CAFFEINE is the most popular stimulant. It is the active chemical found in coffee, tea, and cola drinks, which are often drunk to keep awake or stay alert. Caffeine is also the main ingredient in some pills that you can buy over the counter in drugstores. Heavy users develop symptoms of withdrawal when they stop using caffeine. Scientists are looking into the possibility that excessive use of caffeine can cause benign FIBROUS TUMORS in the breast.

AMPHETAMINES

Not only illegal drugs are abused. One of America's biggest drug problems is the misuse of pills that doctors prescribe. Some of these pills, called AMPHETAMINES (diet pills or "pep" pills like DEXEDRINE and BENZEDRINE), get into the black market or are stolen from the family medicine cabinet. Use of amphetamines, especially when taken without a doctor's supervision, can lead to the well-known yo-yo effect of speed: up one hour and down the next. Amphetamines can make people psychologically dependent and probably cause physical and mental damage when used for a long period of time.

COCAINE

COCAINE ("coke" or "snow"), usually seen in the form of a white powder, comes from the coca bush found in some tropical climates. An illegal drug, cocaine is often smuggled into the United States from South America. Cocaine is usually sniffed into the nostrils, and its stimulant effect comes on quickly.

Cocaine is not addictive, but it can become a habit. Continued use of cocaine can result in severe IRRITATION of membranes in the nostrils, throat, and sinuses. When taken in large doses for a long period of time, cocaine causes SLEEPLESSNESS, ANXIETY, and sometimes DELUSIONS.

Because of its rapid action and powerful stimulant high, cocaine can easily be abused. Because cocaine is very expensive, most users cannot afford to use it in a way that would produce severe dependency. Even so, cocaine use has been increasing in our country. The National Council on Drug Abuse estimates that eight million Americans have tried it at least once and that one million Americans are regular users.

THE DEPRESSANTS

Known as "downers," these drugs DEPRESS the central nervous system, make people SLEEPY, and are dangerous when used in large quantities. There are many drugs in this category, including sedatives (tranquilizers like VALIUM, LIBRIUM, MILTOWN, and BUTISOL) and hypnotics (sleeping pills like NEMBUTAL, SECONAL, DALMANE, and PLACIDYL).

BARBITURATES (AMYTAL, BUTISOL, NEMBUTAL, and SECONAL) are pills prescribed by doctors for a few medical conditions, but they are one of our biggest drug abuse problems. Twice as many people die from overdoses of barbiturates as from overdoses of heroin. Barbiturates (sometimes called "barbs," "downs," or "reds") cause MENTAL CONFUSION, DIZZINESS, and LOSS OF MEMORY. People sometimes get so confused from barbiturates that they forget how many pills they have taken. Often this confusion can result in overdose.

Barbiturates are very ADDICTIVE. In fact, people dependent on barbs have to be very careful coming off them. Sudden withdrawal can cause a medical emergency: extreme RESTLESSNESS, CONVULSIONS, even DEATH. To stop taking barbiturates after using them heavily, talk to a physician first. Barbiturates and alcohol make each other more powerful when taken together. Mixing even a few sleeping pills with alcohol may constitute an overdose and is a frequent cause of accidental death. *Never let anyone take any barbiturates or other downers if they have been drinking.*

OTHER SEDATIVES

People can buy other kinds of depressants, either with a doctor's prescription or over the counter at their pharmacies, that can be taken to help them sleep or to relieve tension.

Minor tranquilizers like VALIUM and LIBRIUM are the

most prescribed drugs in the world, especially for adult women and older men who complain of ANXIETY or DEPRESSION. They are not as dangerous as barbiturates, but all the general cautions about downers still hold. Tranquilizing drugs can create the feeling of needing the drug. People often take them too casually, too often, and too much. Young people show little caution when they take tranquilizers to get high. If you have a prescription for such drugs from your doctor, use them carefully and only as prescribed. Be sure your children understand that these pills are medicines and store them out of the reach of young hands.

THE NARCOTICS

NARCOTICS are like barbiturates. They are derived from OPIUM or are synthesized, and they are all very ADDICTIVE. Used medically as pain-killers, narcotics depress the central nervous system and eventually make people PHYSICALLY and MENTALLY DEPENDENT. CODEINE and DEMEROL are common synthetic narcotics. The OPIATES, a more powerful class of narcotics, are derived directly from the opium poppy and include OPIUM, MORPHINE, and HEROIN. Heroin, usually injected, creates a temporary high and is always addictive if used daily. Although the medical effects of the drug may be no more severe than those of the barbiturates, the great need for heroin often leads to personal desperation, crime, and intense suffering.

THE MIND CHANGERS

HALLUCINOGENS are a class of illegal drugs that have received a great deal of attention in recent years. They act differently in the body from stimulants and depressants. They seem to change the way we see and hear the world around us. They produce HALLUCINATIONS and DELUSIONS.

LSD

Probably the best known mind changer is **LSD** ("acid"). It is one of the most powerful chemicals known; an amount almost too small to see with the naked eye is enough to cause DISORIENTATION for up to twelve hours. Continued used of LSD (Lysergic Acid Diethylamide) can result in serious PERSONALITY BREAKDOWN, although LSD does not create physical dependence.

PCP

A very serious drug of abuse, PHENCYCLIDINE **(PCP),** is a tranquilizer for animals. PCP ("hog" or "angel dust") produces a feeling of NUMBNESS in the arms and legs, and HALLUCINATIONS. Sprinkled on tobacco or marijuana cigarettes or taken in capsules, PCP can create a temporary PSYCHOSIS very much like acute SCHIZOPHRENIA. It often leads to PARANOIA and has been linked with serious violence.

GLUE AND OTHER INHALANTS

Young children sometimes sniff glue and inhale other volatile chemicals, deodorant or hair sprays, or even gasoline fumes to get high. These materials are poisonous and very dangerous. Part of their intoxicating effect comes from their cutting off oxygen to the brain or affecting the lungs. Chemicals in these substances, like the propellant in aerosol, can enter the blood and affect the brain. Overdoses of these chemicals can lead to KIDNEY and BRAIN DAMAGE and DEATH.

Drug abuse is a problem that can be prevented. Prevention is not an easy task, but it is basically a simple one. First, we must understand drugs better. If you or someone you know is headed in a wrong way, talking is not enough. You must take action now, and fast, by getting professional help from your doctor, pharmacist, or Drug Abuse Agency in your community.

ANTIDOTE AND FIRST AID
FOR POISONING

- An emergency **always** exists if someone swallows poison. **Do not delay contacting hospital or physician to obtain advice concerning first aid materials that are not readily available. If necessary, summon police or rescue squad for assistance.** Keep telephone numbers immediately available. Even after emergency measures have been taken, **always** consult physician. A delayed reaction could be fatal.

- It is important to dilute or remove poisons as soon as possible. Keep Syrup of Ipecac (available from most pharmacies or poison centers) in your home to induce vomiting if recommended by physician or indicated on product label. If Syrup of Ipecac is not available, try to make patient vomit by tickling back of throat with finger, spoon, or similar blunt object after giving water.

HOWEVER ...

- Vomiting is **not** recommended in all cases. **Never induce vomiting in a patient who is unconscious or convulsing. Do not induce vomiting if swallowed substance is acidic or corrosive or petroleum distillate products.**

- If poison is from a container, take container with intact label to medical facility treating patient. If poisonous substance is a plant or other unlabeled substance, be prepared to identify suspected substance. Save evidence such as portions of ingested materials from vomitus which may help identify plant or object involved.

The following represent substances most frequently ingested by children, and first aid measures that may be employed **until** medical aid can be summoned.

Substance	Emergency Treatment
MEDICINE (OVERDOSAGE)	
Aspirin and aspirin-containing medications Cough medicine Hormones (including thyroid preparations)	Give 2–3 glasses of water or milk, then induce vomiting UNLESS patient is unconscious or convulsing.

KEEP CALM—DO NOT PANIC—CALL FOR HELP

Substance	Emergency Treatment
Vitamins and iron tablets	Induce vomiting. Then give glass of milk.
Sleeping pills	Induce vomiting. Do **not** induce vomiting or force fluids if patient is unconscious.
Tranquilizers	Induce vomiting unless patient is unconscious. Give 2 tablespoons epsom salts in 2 glasses of water.

HOUSEHOLD CLEANING AND POLISHING AGENTS

Substance	Emergency Treatment
Laundry bleach Automatic dishwasher detergents Household cleaners Furniture polish Cleaning fluid (gasoline, kerosene) Charcoal fire starter	Give 2–3 glasses of milk or water immediately. Do **not** induce vomiting.
Toilet bowl and drain cleaners	Do **not** induce vomiting. Give 2–3 glasses of milk or water at once. **Avoid** gas-forming carbonates and bicarbonates.
Wax remover	Give milk or water. Do **not** induce vomiting.
Fabric softeners	Give milk. Neutralize with **weak** soap (not detergent) solution. Induce vomiting.
Household ammonia	Give citrus juice or diluted (1 tablespoon per glassful) vinegar. Then give 2 raw egg whites or 2 oz. olive oil. Do **not** induce vomiting

INSECTICIDES, POISON SUBSTANCES, PAINTS
(Read labels for content)

Substance	Emergency Treatment
Arsenic	Give glass of milk immediately and induce vomiting. Then give activated charcoal (available from pharmacist).

KEEP CALM—DO NOT PANIC—CALL FOR HELP

Substance	Emergency Treatment
DDT	Induce vomiting. Give 2 tablespoons epsom salts in 2 glasses water.
Lye	Do **not** induce vomiting. Give solution of vinegar (2 tablespoons vinegar in 2 glasses water). Next give 2 raw egg whites or 2 oz. olive oil.
Paint (dry)	Give milk or water. Induce vomiting.
Paint (liquid)	Give 2–3 glasses of milk or water. Do **not** induce vomiting.
COSMETICS Cologne or perfume Hand lotion Liquid makeup Skin lotion After-shave lotion	Give milk. Induce vomiting if large amounts ingested.
Deodorant	Give milk of magnesia. Induce vomiting.
Bubble bath liquid Hair rinse (conditioners) Shampoo	Give milk or water at once. Induce vomiting.
Nail polish and remover Lacquers Bath oil	Give milk. Induce vomiting.
Home permanent neutralizer Permanent wave solution	Give milk or water. Induce vomiting. Then give weak acid such as lemonade, citrus juice, diluted vinegar.
PLANTS **Any** plant is a potential poison.	Induce vomiting if convulsions not imminent. Give artificial respiration if necessary.

KEEP CALM—DO NOT PANIC—CALL FOR HELP

DRUG INTERACTION CHARTS

LIST OF DRUG INTERACTION CHARTS

1. OTC DRUGS
2. ANTIHISTAMINES
3. ANTIDIABETIC DRUGS
4. ANTICOAGULANTS
5. ANTI-PARKINSON DRUGS
6. ORAL CONTRACEPTIVES
7. STEROIDS
8. ANTISPASMODICS
9. HEART MEDICATIONS
10. DIURETICS
11. ANTIHYPERTENSIVES
12. TETRACYCLINES
13. ANTIANXIETY AND SEDATIVES
14. ANTIDEPRESSANTS I
15. ANTIDEPRESSANTS II
16. ANALGESICS
17. CHEMOTHERAPY

Chart 1
OTC DRUGS

ANY OF THESE OTC DRUGS MAY INTERACT WITH

This chart deals strictly with products that can be bought without prescription and points out the potentially hazardous reactions that may occur when they are used in combination.

Over-the-counter (OTC) drugs are effective remedies for many common ailments. You should follow the directions very carefully and never exceed the recommended dose.

You should seek medical advice if the condition you are treating with an OTC product does not clear up or improve within the specified period of time listed on the product. Extended use of products beyond the recommended time may mask the symptoms of a more serious problem that requires treatment by your physician.

When selecting a product for a cold or cough, it is advisable to check with your physician or pharmacist and to mention other household remedies or prescription medications you are taking.

OTC products that interact with prescription and other medications and substances are described in the following charts.

Alcoholic beverages
Cheracol and Cheracol D
Cosanyl-DM
Creo-Terpin
Demazin
Dristan Cough Formula
Novahistine products
Nyquil
Pertussin
Robitussin products
Triaminic products
Valadol Liquid
Vicks Formula 44 and 44D

ANY OF THESE OTC/FOOD ITEMS		AND RESULT IN THESE INTERACTIONS

Alka-Seltzer products	4-Way cold products	Different interactions may occur depending upon the combinations of column 1 and column 2 OTC medications.
Alka-2	Measurin	
Allerest	Midol	
Anacin products	Neo-Synephrine products	
A. R. M.		1. If you combine a cough or cold product that contains alcohol from column 1 with a pain or fever product from column 2, the combination could result in irritation to your stomach lining and nausea could occur.
Arthritis Strength Bufferin	Novahistine products	
A. S. A. Enseals and A. S. A. Compound	Nyquil	
	Nytol	
Ascriptin products	PAC	
	Pamprin	
Aspergum	Robitussin products	2. If you combine a cough or cold product containing alcohol from column 1 with a cold or allergy medication containing an antihistamine from column 2, you may experience excessive drowsiness and a decrease in mental alertness.
Aspirin (all brands)	Sinutab	
Bayer products	Sleep-Eze	
Bufferin	*Sodium Salicylate	
Cama	Sominex	
Chlorpheniramine products	Sudafed	
	Triaminic products	
Chlor-Trimeton products	Triaminicin products	3. Combining cough or cold remedies from either column could compound the problems of drowsiness and mental alertness. Always read the label carefully and if you have any questions check with your pharmacist or physician.
Compoz	Triaminicol	
Comtrex	Vanquish	
Contac	Vicks Formula 44 and 44D	
Conar		
Coricidin products		
Coryban-D		
Demazin		
Dormin		
Ecotrin		
Empirin		
Exedrin		

*generic drug—available without prescription upon request to pharmacist

Chart 2
ANTIHISTAMINES

ANY OF THESE Rx DRUGS
MAY INTERACT WITH

The drugs listed in column 1 are antihistamines and antihistamine combinations. There are many different types of antihistamines available for your physician's use. Some common types are used for runny nose, watery eyes, and other ailments caused by the common cold or allergies. Other types of antihistamines are used in the treatment of nausea, vomiting, dizziness, motion sickness, or itching. Sometimes antihistamines are prescribed for insomnia because they cause drowsiness.

Use of antihistamines may cause dryness of the mouth and throat. This may be relieved by chewing gum or sucking hard candy. Smoking tends to cause further irritation and should be avoided.

If stomach upset occurs while taking one of these medications, try taking it with food or milk, or immediately after meals, according to your doctor's directions.

Azatidine (Optimine)
Brompheniramine (Dimetane)
Chlorpheniramine maleate
 (Teldrin)
Clemastine (Tavist)
Cyproheptadine (Periactin)
Dexchlorpheniramine
 (Polaramine)
Dimetapp
Diphenhydramine (Benadryl)
Disophrol
Drixoral
Naldecon
Nolamine
Novafed A
Orande
Promethazine (Phenergan)
Tripelennamine
 (Pyribenzamine)
Triprolidine (Actidil)

ANY OF THESE OTC/FOOD ITEMS	AND RESULT IN THESE INTERACTIONS
Alcoholic beverages Allerest A.R.M. Bayer Decongestant Cheracol and Cheracol D Chlor-Trimeton Compoz Comtrex Conar Contac Coricidin products Coryban-D Cossanyl DM Creo-Terpin Demazin Dormin Dristan products Neo-Synephrine products Novahistine products Nyquil Nytol Penetro Pertussin Robitussin products Sinutab Sleep-Eze Sominex Super Anahist Triaminicin products Triaminicol Vicks Sinex Vicks Formula 44 and 44D	Unless otherwise advised by your physician, you should avoid combining any of the drugs in column 1 with any of the OTC products in column 2. A combination of these products could result in drowsiness, dizziness, and a decrease in mental alertness. If these medications must be combined, extra caution should be exercised while driving or operating any machinery.

Chart 3
ANTIDIABETIC DRUGS

ANY OF THESE **Rx** DRUGS
MAY INTERACT WITH

The medications listed in column 1 are referred to as antidiabetic or hypoglycemic agents. They are often prescribed to aid the diabetic patient in the storage and utilization of sugar. Injectable insulin may be affected by the interactions listed and by other OTC and Rx drugs.

Some mild side effects may be noticed when first taking these drugs: loss of appetite, nausea, stomach upset. These symptoms usually disappear in a few weeks. Prolonged discomfort should be reported to your doctor, as should a persistent sore throat, low fever, diarrhea, or dark urine.

Follow your doctor's directions closely and never take extra tablets or increase your insulin dosage without his or her consent.

The major offending OTC interactions involve cough or cold preparations.

Acetohexamide (Dymelor)
Chlorpropamide (Diabinese)
Insulin
Tolbutamide (Orinase)
Tolazamide (Tolinase)

ANY OF THESE OTC/FOOD ITEMS		AND RESULT IN THESE INTERACTIONS
Alcoholic beverages	Neo-Synephrine products	Alcoholic beverages or OTC products containing alcohol may cause either an increase or decrease in your blood sugar level. You should avoid using these products unless otherwise directed by your physician.
Alka-Seltzer products	Novahistine products	
Alka-2	Nyquil	
Anacin products	PAC	
Bufferin	Pamprin	
A.S.A. Enseals and A.S.A. Compound	Pepto-Bismol	
	Pertussin	Aspirin-containing products could cause a lowering in your blood sugar level when combined with your antidiabetic medication or insulin. Close monitoring of your sugar level is recommended if you must take an aspirin-containing product.
Ascriptin products	Robitussin products	
Aspergum	*Sodium Salicylate	
Aspirin (all brands)	Sominex	
Bayer products	Super Anahist	
Cama	Triaminic products	
Cheracol and Cheracol D	Triaminicin products	
Coricidin products	Vanquish	
Coryban-D	Vicks Formula 44 and 44D	
Cosanyl-DM		
Creo-Terpin		
Demazin		
Dristan products		
Ecotrin		
Empirin		
Excedrin		
4-Way cold products		
Gemnisyn		
Measurin		
Midol		

*generic drug—available without prescription upon request to pharmacist

Chart 4
ANTICOAGULANTS

ANY OF THESE Rx DRUGS
MAY INTERACT WITH

The medications in column 1 are known as anticoagulant drugs (blood thinners). They are mainly used to reduce the probability of the formation of blood clots in the circulatory system.

Frequent checkups by your doctor are necessary to test the clotting time ("pro time") of your blood. Your doctor will adjust your prescription based on the results of these tests. If you change doctors or visit a dentist, alert him or her to the type and strength of the anticoagulant you are taking. Never take another prescription medication without the consent of your doctor. Too much anticoagulant (or anticoagulants mixed with certain drugs) may cause unusual bleeding. Notify your doctor if you notice any of the following symptoms: prolonged or excessive bleeding from nose, gums, cuts, or scrapes; red in the urine or black stools; vomiting or coughing blood; prolonged headaches; abdominal pain; unusual discharge during menstruation; prolonged diarrhea; fever; or loss of appetite.

In the use of anticoagulants, it is *not* advisable to change to a generic equivalent unless directed by your doctor. Inform your doctor if you become pregnant or are nursing.

Acenocoumarol (Sintrom)
Anisinione (Miradon)
Bishydroxycoumarin
  (Dicumarol)
Phenindione (Hedulin)
Phenprocoumon (Liquamar)
Warfarin Sodium (Coumadin)

ANY OF THESE OTC/FOOD ITEMS	AND RESULT IN THESE INTERACTIONS
Aspirin (all brands) *Soldium Salicylate Alka-2 Sominex Alka-Seltzer Super Anahist products Triaminicin A.P.C. products Arthritis Strength Vanquish Bufferin A.S.A. Enseals and A.S.A. Compound Ascription products Aspergum Bayer products Bufferin Cama Coricidin products Dristan products Ecotrin Empirin Excedrin 4-Way cold products Gemnisyn Measurin Midol PAC Pamprin	The OTC drugs listed could increase the activity of your Rx medication and lead to excessive bleeding. The foods listed are high in vitamin K and could reduce the effectiveness of your anticoagulant drug.

Leafy green vegetables, such as cabbage, spinach, kale, alfalfa. Other vegetables, such as cauliflower

*generic drug—available without prescription upon request to pharmacist

Chart 5
ANTI-PARKINSON DRUGS

ANY OF THESE Rx DRUGS
MAY INTERACT WITH

The medications listed in chapter 5 are referred to as anti-Parkinson agents. These drugs are used in the control of involuntary movements associated with various disorders. Alert your physician if you have a history of peptic ulcers, are pregnant, or are nursing.

If you require a vitamin supplement while taking this medication, your physician can select a product that does not contain vitamin B-6. The foods listed in the interaction chart contain higher amounts of B-6 and should be avoided when possible.

Levodopa (Bendopa, Dopar, Larodopa)
Sinemet (Levadopa and Carbidopa)

ANY OF THESE OTC/FOOD ITEMS	AND RESULT IN THESE INTERACTIONS

Products containing vitamin B-6 (Pyridoxine), such as:
   Allbee products
   B Complex products
   Beminal products
   Hexa-Betalin
   Orexin Softab Tablets
   Stresstabs 600, Stresscaps
   Trophite
   Vio-Bec
 	
Foods containing large amounts of vitamin B-6, such as:
   corn
   liver
   yeast
	The combination of the OTC products in column 2 with your anti-Parkinson medication could severely decrease its effectiveness.
	
	The food products listed could also result in a decreased effectiveness of your Rx medication, depending on your dietary consumption.

Chart 6
ORAL CONTRACEPTIVES

ANY OF THESE Rx DRUGS
MAY INTERACT WITH

The drugs listed in column 1 are oral contraceptives. There are many different types and strengths of oral contraceptives that allow your physician to select for you the best pill with the least number of side effects.

Women who take oral contraceptives should be aware of the increased risk of side effects involving the heart and blood vessels.

Follow directions closely. Report any unusual swelling, rash, yellowing of the skin or eyes, or pains in the chest muscles or abdomen to your physician. He or she may be able to eliminate some of these side effects by changing the dose or strength of your medication.

Maintain an adequate diet since these drugs can reduce your vitamin B-6 and C levels. If you must reduce your caloric intake, an OTC vitamin B complex and C should be added.

Brevicon
Demulen
Enovid and Enovid-E
Loestrin
Modicon
Norinyl
Norlestrin
Ortho-Novum
Ovcon
Ovral
Ovulen

ANY OF THESE OTC/FOOD ITEMS		AND RESULT IN THESE INTERACTIONS
Cyanocobalamin (vitamin B-12) Folic Acid Pyridoxine (vitamin B-6) Vitamin E	Theragram products	The top group of vitamin products may be depleted when taking oral contraceptives. Supplementing your diet with an OTC product containing these ingredients may be advisable.
Vitamin A-containing products, such as: Cod Liver Oil Mi-Cebrin Myadec Optilets-500 and Optilets-M-500 Super D Perles		The lower group of products containing vitamin A, if taken in excess, could lead to an excessive accumulation of vitamin A while on oral contraceptives.

Chart 7
STEROIDS

ANY OF THESE Rx DRUGS
MAY INTERACT WITH

The medications listed in column 1 are referred to as steroids. Steroids differ widely in their medical usage, and there are many types available. Your physician will choose the type best suited to you.

Steroids are prescribed often for arthritic, allergic, skin, breathing, hormonal, and eye disorders. Steroids are sometimes used for short courses of treatment. When used over a long period of time, frequent check-ups by your doctor are advised. Never take a steroid medication longer than your physician directs.

When taking this medication you should try to avoid stressful situations. Inform your doctor if you have a history of ulcers. Inform your doctor of any other medication you are taking and if you become pregnant or are nursing.

Notify your physician if you notice persistent thirst, frequent urination, or blurred vision. *While on these medications you should not receive any vaccinations or undergo any surgical procedure without checking with your doctor first.*

Betamethasone (Celestone)
Cortisone (Cortone)
Dexamethasone (Decadron, Hexadrol)
Fludrocortisone (Florinef)
Hydrocortisone (Cortef, Hydrocortone)
Methylprednisolone (Medrol)
Prednisolone (Delta-Cortef)
Prednisone (Deltasone, Meticorten)
Triamcinolone (Aristocort, Kenacort)

ANY OF THESE OTC/FOOD ITEMS		AND RESULT IN THESE INTERACTIONS

Alcoholic beverages and products containing alcohol	Empirin	The combination of any of the OTC remedies in column 2 with your steroid medication could result in an increased potential for nausea, vomiting, ulceration, or damage to the stomach lining. Unless otherwise directed by your physician, you should not combine these drugs.
Alka-Seltzer products	Exedrin	
Alka-2	4-Way cold products	
Allerest	Gemnisyn	
Anacin products	Measurin	
Arthritis Strength Bufferin	Midol	
A.S.A. Enseals and A.S.A. Compound	Neo-Synephrine products	A decrease in your steroid's effectiveness could also result from combining them with these OTC products.
Ascriptin products	Novahistine products	
Aspergum	Nyquil	
Aspirin (all brands)	Nytol	
Bayer products	PAC	
Bufferin	Pamprin	
Cama	Robitussin products	
Chlorpheniramine products	Sinutab	
Chlor-Trimeton products	Sleep-Eze	
Compoz	*Sodium Salicylate	
Contac	Sominex	
Conar	Sudafed	
Coricidin products	Triaminic products	
Coryban-D	Triaminicin products	
Demazin	Triaminicol	
Dormin	Vanquish	
Ecotrin	Vicks Formula 44 and 44D	

Alcoholic beverages and products containing alcohol
Alka-Seltzer products
Alka-2
Allerest
Anacin products
Arthritis Strength Bufferin
A.S.A. Enseals and A.S.A. Compound
Ascriptin products
Aspergum
Aspirin (all brands)
Bayer products
Bufferin
Cama
Chlorpheniramine products
Chlor-Trimeton products
Compoz
Contac
Conar
Coricidin products
Coryban-D
Demazin
Dormin
Ecotrin

Empirin
Exedrin
4-Way cold products
Gemnisyn
Measurin
Midol
Neo-Synephrine products
Novahistine products
Nyquil
Nytol
PAC
Pamprin
Robitussin products
Sinutab
Sleep-Eze
*Sodium Salicylate
Sominex
Sudafed
Triaminic products
Triaminicin products
Triaminicol
Vanquish
Vicks Formula 44 and 44D

The combination of any of the OTC remedies in column 2 with your steroid medication could result in an increased potential for nausea, vomiting, ulceration, or damage to the stomach lining. Unless otherwise directed by your physician, you should not combine these drugs.

A decrease in your steroid's effectiveness could also result from combining them with these OTC products.

*generic drug—available without prescription upon request to pharmacist

Chart 8
ANTISPASMODICS

ANY OF THESE Rx DRUGS
MAY INTERACT WITH

The medications listed in chapter 8 are referred to as antispasmodics. They are used primarily for disorders of the stomach but may be used also in treating certain types of urinary, kidney, or allergic disorders.

The medications may cause drowsiness, dizziness, or blurring of vision. Exercise caution if driving or involved in any activity requiring mental alertness. Dryness of the mouth may occur and may be relieved by chewing gum or candy. If the dryness persists, or if you notice a skin rash, flushing, or eye pain, notify your physician.

These medications may decrease perspiration, which could lead to fever or possibly heat stroke. If you notice a slight fever developing, remain in a cool environment.

If you are taking antacids while on this medication, allow an hour or two between the two medications. They should not be taken at the same time.

Atropine preparations
Belladonna preparations
Benztropin Mesylate
  (Cogentin)
Dicyclomine (Bentyl)
Glycopyrrolate (Robinul)
Librax
Propantheline (Pro-Banthine)
Trihexyphenidyl (Artane)

ANY OF THESE OTC/FOOD ITEMS	AND RESULT IN THESE INTERACTIONS
Alcoholic Beverages Vicks Formula 44 and 44D Allerest A.R.M. Bayer Decongestant Chlorpheniramine products Chlor-Trimeton products Compoz Comtrex Conar Contac Coricidin products Coryban D Demazin Dormin Dristan products Neo-Synephrine products Novahistine products Nyquil Nytol Pyrilamine Robitussin products Sinutab Sleep-Eze Sominex Super Anahist Triaminic products Triaminicin products Triaminicol Vicks Sinex	The combination of any of the OTC products in column 2 with any of the prescription medications could compound the problem of mouth dryness. A possibility of blurred vision, drowsiness, or a decrease in mental alertness may arise if you combine an antispasmodic with any of the OTC products listed.

Chart 9
HEART MEDICATIONS

ANY OF THESE Rx DRUGS
MAY INTERACT WITH

The medications listed in column 1 are commonly referred to as heart medications. They are prescribed to help the heart pump more effectively. It is important to follow your doctor's directions closely and never to take extra heart medication. Try not to miss a dose and take your medicine at the same time every day.

Notify your doctor if you notice any of the following problems while taking your medication: unexplained loss of appetite, weakness, fatigue, shortness of breath; prolonged nausea, vomiting, abdominal pain, diarrhea; blurred vision, yellow or green halos around objects.

These medications are usually prescribed for long-term use. It is important that you have regular check-ups so that your doctor can adjust the dosage or strength of the medication if necessary.

Digifortis
Digitoxin (Crystodigin, Purodigin)
Digoxin (Lanoxin)
Gitalin (Gitaligin)

ANY OF THESE OTC/FOOD ITEMS	AND RESULT IN THESE INTERACTIONS

Aludrox   Mylanta
*Aluminum   products
  Hydroxide
  products
Amphojel
Ascriptin and
  Ascriptin AID
Camalox
Dristan
Gelusil products
Kaolin/Pectin
  (Kaopectate)
Maalox products
*Magnesium
  Hydroxide
  products
*Magnesium Tris-
  ilicate products
Milk of
  Magnesia
	The first group of OTC prod-
	ucts may decrease the effec-
	tiveness of your heart medica-
	tion if taken at the same time.
	Unless otherwise directed by
	your physician, take any of
	these OTC products at least 2
	to 4 hours after your heart pill.

AsthmaNefrin   Va-Trol-Nol
Breatheasy
Bronkaid
  products
*Epinephrine
  (Adrenaline)
Medihaler-EPI
Primatene Mist
Vaponefrin
  Solution
	The second group of OTC
	antiasthmatic products could
	produce irregular heart beats if
	taken with heart medication.
	Check with your physician
	before using them.

*generic drug—available without
prescription upon request to
pharmacist

Chart 10
DIURETICS

ANY OF THESE Rx DRUGS
MAY INTERACT WITH

The drugs listed in column 1 are collectively referred to as diuretics or high blood pressure drugs. There are many different types from which your doctor can select the most appropriate for your condition. The drugs work by aiding the kidney to increase the production of urine and rid the body of excess water and fluids.

These drugs are used to treat high blood pressure, swelling, certain heart conditions, and water retention. Some are used in the treatment of glaucoma.

Since the diuretics may cause a loss of potassium, your doctor may advise you to drink fruit juices or eat bananas to replenish the body's loss of this mineral. He may give you a potassium-replacement drug if necessary. Notify him if you notice any weakness, fatigue, rash, diarrhea, or joint or foot pain.

Spironolactone (Aldactone, Aldactazide) and Triamterene (Dyazide, Dyrenium) are used to conserve the loss of potassium, and supplements may not be necessary or may even be harmful.

Acetazolamide (Diamox)
Bendroflumethiazide
 (Naturetin)
Benthiazide (Exna)
Chlorothiazide (Diuril)
Chlorthalidone (Hygroton)
Dichlorphenamide (Daranide)
Ethacrynic Acid (Edecrin)
Ethoxzolamide (Cardrase,
 Ethamide)
Furosemide (Lasix)
Hydrochlorthiazide (Esidrix,
 HydroDiuril)
Methazolamide (Neptazane)
Methyclothiazide (Enduron)
Metolazone (Diulo,
 Zaroxolyn)
Polythiazide (Renese)
Quinethazone (Hydromox)
Trichlormethiazide (Metahydrin, Naqua)

ANY OF THESE OTC/FOOD ITEMS		AND RESULT IN THESE INTERACTIONS

Afrinol	Nyquil	The alcohol-containing OTC products, when combined with a prescription product in column 1, could cause severe drowsiness, dizziness, and a decrease in mental alertness. Caution should be exercised if you drive or operate machinery and must combine these drugs.
Alcoholic beverages	Ornacol products	
Alconefrin	Ornex	
Allerest products	Orthoxicol	
A.R.M.	Primatene Mist	
AsthmaNefrin	Privine	
Bayer Decongestant	Phenylephrine products	
Breatheasy	Phenylpropanol-amine products	The OTC cold remedies (decongestants) listed could lead to an increase in your blood pressure when combined with your diuretic. Check with your physician before using these products.
Bromo Quinine cold tablets	Romilar products	
Bronkaid products	Sinutab	
Caffeine	Sudafed	
Cheracol and Cheracol D	Super Anahist	
Contac	Triaminic products	
Coricidin products	Triaminicol	
Coryban-D	Trind and Trind-DM	
Cosanyl DM	Ursinus	
DayCare	Va-Tro-Nol	
Demazine	Vicks Inhaler	
Dimacol products	4-Way Cold Tablets and Spray	
Dristan products		
*Epinephrine (Adrenaline)		
Fedrazil		
Medihaler-Epi		
Neo-Synephrine products (Phenylephrine HCL)		
Nodoz		
Novahistine products		

*generic drug—available without prescription upon request to pharmacist

Chart 11
ANTIHYPERTENSIVES

ANY OF THESE RX DRUGS
MAY INTERACT WITH

The medications listed in column 1 are referred to as antihypertensives and are used in the treatment of high blood pressure. Some of these drugs may cause dizziness or drowsiness upon initial therapy. Therefore, avoid sudden changes in posture and balance.

Normally if your medication is changed or discontinued, it should be gradually reduced over a period of days.

Notify your physician if you notice swelling, fever, fatigue, chills, troubled breathing, sore throat, diarrhea, or fast heart rate.

Appendix 10 contains diuretics which are also used to treat blood pressure.

Guanethidine
  (Esimil, Ismelin)
Hydralazine
  (Apresazide, Apresoline)
Methyldopa
  (Aldomet, Aldoril, Aldoclor)
Reserpine
  (Serpasil, Reserpoid)
Reserpine Combinations
  Demi-Regroton
  Diupres
  Diutensin-R
  Exna-R
  Hydropres
  Hydroserpine
  Metatensin
  Naquival
  Regroton
  Salutensin
  Ser-Ap-Es

ANY OF THESE OTC/FOOD ITEMS		AND RESULT IN THESE INTERACTIONS
A.R.M.	*Phenylephrine products	Combining alcohol-containing OTC products with antihypertensives could result in severe drowsiness and a decrease in mental alertness.
Afrinol		
Alconefrin	*Phenylpropanolamine products	
Allerest products		
AsthmaNefrin	Romilar products	
Bayer Decongestant	Sinutab	
	Sudafed	Combining antihypertensives with cough or cold remedies containing a decongestant could result in an unpredictable increase or decrease in your blood pressure. Check with your physician before combining these products with antihypertensives.
Breatheasy	Super Anahist	
BromoQuinine Cold Tablets	Triaminic products	
Bronkaid products	Triaminicol	
Cheracol and Cheracol D	Trind and Trind-DM	
Comtrex	Ursinus	
Contac	Va-Tro-Nol	
Coricidin products	Vicks Sinex	
Cosanyl DM	4-Way Cold products	
DayCare	OTC Diet Aids, e.g., Dex-a-trim, Dietac	
Demazin		
Dimacol products		
Dristan products		
*Epinephrine (Adrenaline)		
Fedrazil		
Medihaler-Epi		
Neo-Synephrine products		
Nodoz		
Nyquil		
Ornacol products		
Ornex		
Orthoxicol		
Primatene Mist		
Privine		

*generic drug—available without prescription upon request to pharmacist

Chart 12
TETRACYCLINES

ANY OF THESE Rx DRUGS
MAY INTERACT WITH

The drugs listed in column 1 are referred to as the *tetracyclines*. These antibiotics are used for both long and short-term infections. Different forms of tetracycline allow your physician to select the appropriate type for your particular illness.

The tetracyclines can cause your skin to be more sensitive to the burning rays of the sun. If you are going to be in the sun, use a sunscreen agent for protection.

Avoid these medications if you are nursing or become pregnant. They should also be avoided by infants and young children since damage to the tooth enamel or discoloration of the teeth may result from their use.

The best time to take these drugs is one hour before a meal or two hours after, unless otherwise directed. They should be taken with water.

Be sure to take all of your medication, even if you feel better in a few days. If discontinued too soon, your condition may recur.

If you notice a skin rash or develop severe diarrhea, notify your physician.

Achromycin and Achromycin V
Achrostatin V
Bristacycline
Cyclopar
Kesso-Tetra
Mysteclin-F
Panmycin
Robitet
SK-Tetracycline
Sumycin
Tetrachel
Tetracine
Tetracyn
Tetrex

ANY OF THESE OTC/FOOD ITEMS	AND RESULT IN THESE INTERACTIONS
Iron preparations (Fer-In-Sol products, Ferrous Sulfate tablets) Vanquish	The combination of any of the OTC products or food items listed in column 2 with any of the antibiotics in column 1 can cause a decrease in the effectiveness of the antibiotic.
Milk and dairy products Antacids and products containing any of the following ingredients in any form: calcium, aluminum, magnesium.	Unless otherwise directed by your physician, take your antibiotic at least one hour before or two hours after a meal, as directed.
Alka-2 Alka-Seltzer products Aludrox Amphojel Ascriptin and Ascriptin AID Bufferin Cama Camalox Creamalin Dicarbosil Di-Gel Dristan products Gelusil Maalox products Milk of Magnesia Mylanta products Titralac Triaminicin products Tums	

Chart 13

ANTIANXIETY DRUGS AND SEDATIVES

ANY OF THESE Rx DRUGS
MAY INTERACT WITH

The medications listed in column 1 are a combination of drug groups ranging from antianxiety, sedative, and hypnotic to antypsychotic medications. They are used to treat various ailments from nervousness and anxiety to muscle tension, nausea, vomiting, insomnia, itching, hives, and skin rash. Anticonvulsant or epilepsy medications may interact in the same manner as those listed. These medications should be used only as directed; overuse may be habit-forming. It is extremely important to follow directions closely and never take additional doses. If you are taking a sleeping medication listed in this appendix, try to avoid using it on a daily basis unless otherwise directed.

Inform your doctor if you notice any of the following: excessive drowsiness, fatigue, difficulty in concentrating, dizziness, nightmares, irritability, or muscular spasms.

It is extremely important not to mix any of the medications in column 1 unless directed by your doctor. Combining drugs in this fashion may enhance the depression of the nervous system. Inform your doctor if you become pregnant or are nursing.

Amobarbital (Amytal)
Chloral Hydrate (Noctec)
Chlordiazepoxide (Librium, Limbitrol)
Chlorpromazine (Thorazine)
Clonazepam (Clonopin)
Clorazepate (Tranxene, Azene)
Diazepam (Valium)
Ethchlorvynol (Placidyl)
Fluphenazine (Prolixin)
Flurazepam (Dalmane)
Glutethimide (Doriden)
Hydroxyzine (Atarax, Vistaril)
Lorazepam (Ativan)
Meprobamate (Equanil, Miltown)
Oxazepam (Serax)
Pentobarbital (Nembutal)
Perphenazine (Trilafon)
Phenobarbital (Luminal)
Prazepam (Centrax)
Prochlorperazine (Compazine)
Promazine (Sparine)
Secobarbital (Seconal, Tuinal)
Triclofos (Triclos)
Trifluoperazine (Stelazine)
Thioridazine (Mellaril)
Thiothixene (Navane)

ANY OF THESE OTC/FOOD ITEMS	AND RESULT IN THESE INTERACTIONS
Alcoholic beverages or products containing alcohol Allerest A.R.M. Bayer Decongestant Cheracol and Cheracol D Coldene Compoz Comtrex Conar Contac Coricidin products Coryban-D Cosanyl DM Creo-Terpin Demazin Dormin Dristan products Neo-Synephrine products Novahistine products Nyquil Nytol Pertussin Robitussin products Sinutab Sleep-Eze Sominex Super Anahist Triaminicin products Triaminicol Vicks Formula 44 and 44D Vicks Sinex	Combining any of the antianxiety or sedative prescription products in column 1 with any of the OTC products listed in column 2 would result in severe drowsiness, dizziness, nausea, and decreased mental alertness. A possible increase in depression of the central nervous system could also occur. Unless otherwise directed by your physician, these combinations should be avoided.

Chart 14
ANTIDEPRESSANTS I

ANY OF THESE Rx DRUGS
MAY INTERACT WITH

The medications listed in Appendix 14 are referred to as antidepressants. Some may also be prescribed for anxiety and for some childhood disorders.

These drugs often require up to four weeks of therapy before there is a noticeable improvement in your condition. Therefore, be sure to continue the medication even if you feel it does not benefit you. In the first weeks of therapy you may experience drowsiness or dryness of mouth. These symptoms should improve after a few weeks; do not discontinue the medication without your doctor's consent. Abrupt withdrawal may cause nausea and headache.

These drugs sometimes cause drowsiness and blurred vision—be cautious when driving or performing other activities requiring mental alertness. Use extra protection in the sun; these drugs may cause you to burn more easily. They should be used with extreme caution in persons with or having predisposition to glaucoma. Notify physician if unexplainable sore throat occurs.

Amitriptyline (Elavil, Endep)
Amoxapine (Asendin)
Cyclobenzaprine (Flexeril)
Desipramine (Norpramin, Pertofrane)
Doxepin (Adapin, Sinequan)
Etrafon
Imipramine (Tofranil)
Limbitrol
Maprotiline (Ludiomil)
Nortriptyline (Aventyl, Pamelor)
Triavil
Triimipramine (Surmontil)

ANY OF THESE OTC/FOOD ITEMS		AND RESULT IN THESE INTERACTIONS
Alcoholic beverages and products containing alcohol	Vicks Formula 44 and 44D Vicks Sinex	The combination of any of these prescription drugs in column 1 with the OTC products listed could result in severe drowsiness, dizziness, nausea, and decreased mental alertness.
Allerest A.R.M. Bayer Decongestant		Increased depression of the central nervousness system could also occur if these groups of drugs are combined.
Cheracol and Cheracol D Compoz Comtrex Conar Contac Coricidin products Coryban-D Cosanyl DM Creo-Terpin Demazin Dormin Dristan products Neo-Synephrine products Novahistine products Nyquil Nytol Pertussin Robitussin products Sinutab Sleep-Eze Sominex Super Anahist Triaminicin products Triaminicol		Check with your physician before combining any of these antidepressants and OTC products. The prescription drugs in column 1, Appendix 13, could also cause these interactions if combined with these antidepressants.

Chart 15
ANTIDEPRESSANTS II

**ANY OF THESE Rx DRUGS
MAY INTERACT WITH**

The medications listed in column 1 are referred to as M.A.O. (monamine oxidase) inhibitors. They are prescribed for treatment of depression, anxiety, and other medical disorders.

These are very potent drugs, and special precautions should be followed. *Do not* discontinue the medication unless so directed by your physician. You may notice dizziness, drowsiness, weakness, or blurred vision upon starting this medication. If these symptoms persist, notify your doctor. Also, you should notify your doctor if you develop severe headaches, skin rash, darkening of the urine, yellowing of the skin, persistent headaches, sore throat, or diarrhea.

It is of utmost importance to avoid the interacting foods and OTC medications listed here while taking this medication, and for at least 2 weeks after.

Furazolidone (Furoxone)
Isocarboxazid (Marplan)
Pargyline (Eutonyl)
Phenelzine (Nardil)
Procarbazine (Matulane)
Tranylcypromine (Parnate)

ANY OF THESE OTC/FOOD ITEMS		AND RESULT IN THESE INTERACTIONS

Cheeses	Summer Sausage, Pepperoni	The combination of any OTC drug products or foods in column 2 with any of the Rx medications in column 1 could result in *severe* hypertension (high blood pressure).
Cheddar		
Emmenthaler	Red Wines	
Gruyere	Bananas	
Stilton	Figs	
Brie	Avocados	
Camembert	Fava	A combination of this type could also result in fever and excitement and possibly lead to convulsions.
Chocolate	Yeast Extract	
Coffee	Chicken Liver	
Cola	Beef Liver	
Fermented	OTC Diet Aids,	
Sausages,	e.g., Dex-a-trim,	It is important to always check with your pharmacist or physician before taking any OTC item while on the prescription medications in column 1.
fermented Bolognas, Salamis,	Dietac	

A.R.M.	Dimacol
Adrenaline	Dristan products
Afrinol	*Epinephrine (Adrenaline)
Alcoholic beverages or products containing alcohol	Fedrazil
	Medihaler-Epi
	Neo-Synephrine products
Alconefrin	Nodoz
Allerest	Nyquil
AsthmaNefrin	Ornacol products
Bayer Decongestant	Ornex
Breatheasy	Orthoxicol
Bronkaid products	Primatene Mist
Cheracol and Cheracol D	Privine
	Phenylephrine preparations
Comtrex	Phenylpropanolamine preparations
Contac	
Coricidin products	Romilar products
Cosanyl DM	Sinutab
DayCare	Sudafed
Demazin	

Super Anahist	Ursinus
Triaminic products	Va-Tro-Nol Drops
Triaminicol	Vicks Sinex
Trind and Trind-DM	4-Way cold products

*generic drug—available without prescription upon request to pharmacist

Chart 16
ANALGESICS

ANY OF THESE Rx DRUGS
MAY INTERACT WITH

The analgesics referred to in this section are used in the treatment of arthritis, cramps, muscular aches and pains, and headaches. They work by relieving inflammation, swelling, stiffness, and pain.

Propoxyphene (Darvon, Darvocet) and codeine-containing products can also react similarly with these OTC drug products.

These medications should be taken with food or milk to offset possible stomach distress.

Notify your doctor if you have a history of allergic reaction to aspirin, ulcers, or bleeding problems; or if you notice skin rash, itching, ringing in the ears, blurred vision, swelling, or unusual weight gain. Slight dizziness may occur when first beginning these drugs.

Do not take these medications with alcoholic beverages.

Fenoprofen (Nalfon)
Ibuprofen (Motrin)
Indomethacin (Indocin)
Meclofenamate (Meclomin)
Naproxen (Anaprox, Naprosyn)
Oxyphenbutazone (Oxalid, Tandearil)
Phenylbutazone (Azolid, Butazolidin)
Sulindac (Clinoril)
Zomepirac (Zomax)

ANY OF THESE OTC/FOOD ITEMS		AND RESULT IN THESE INTERACTIONS
Alcoholic beverages	Novahistine products	OTC alcohol-containing products and alcoholic beverages when combined with the analgesics listed in column 1 may result in nausea or stomach distress. If both these medications have to be taken, it would be advisable not to take them at the same time.
Alka-Seltzer	Nyquil	
Alka-2	PAC	
Anacin products	Pamprin	
A.S.A. and A.S.A. Compound	Pepto-Bismol	
	Pertussin	
Ascriptin products	Robitussin products	Other OTC preparations listed in column 2 are those that contain aspirin or salicylates. If these products are combined with the analgesics in column 1, a possible decrease in the effectiveness of your prescription analgesic may occur.
Aspergum	*Sodium Salicylate	
Aspirin (all brands)		
	Sominex	
Bayer products	Super Anahist	
Bufferin	Triaminic products	
Cama		
Cheracol and Cheracol D	Triaminicin products	
Coricidin products	Vanquish	
	Vicks Formula 44 and 44D	
Coryban-D		
Cosanyl-DM		
Creo-Terpin		
Demazin		
Dristan products		
Ecotrin		
Empirin		
Excedrin		
4-Way cold products		
Gemnisyn		
Measurin		
Midol		
Neo-Synephrine products		

*generic drug—available without prescription upon request to pharmacist

Chart 17
CHEMOTHERAPY

ANY OF THESE Rx DRUGS
MAY INTERACT TITH

The antineoplastic drugs listed in the following charts are primarily used to aid in the treatment of various forms of cancer. Some of the drugs listed are also used for other medical disorders, e.g., psoriasis.

Strict adherence to your doctor's directions and frequent check-ups will aid in avoiding adverse side effects. Alcoholic beverages should be avoided while taking these medications.

Nursing or pregnancy should be avoided for at least eight weeks after therapy. One should avoid stressful situations and maintain a well-balanced diet.

Notify your doctor if you notice persistent diarrhea, fever, chills, sore throat, unusual bleeding, bruising, yellowing of the eyes or skin.

Fluorouracil (5-Fu)

Methotrexate

ANY OF THESE OTC/FOOD ITEMS	AND RESULT IN THESE INTERACTIONS
Acidic foods, such as orange juice	If 5-Fu is used orally, acidic foods such as orange juice, if taken at the same time, could decrease its effectiveness.
Alka-2 Alka-Seltzer products Anacin products Arthritis Strength Bufferin A.S.A. Compound Ascriptin products Aspergum Aspirin (all brands) Bayer products Bufferin Cama Coricidin products Dristan products Ecotrin Empirin Excedrin 4-Way cold products Measurin Midol PAC Pamprin Pepto-Bismol *Sodium Salicylate Sominex Super Anahist Triaminicin products Vanquish	The second group of products should be avoided with Methotrexate because they could increase the toxic effects of methotrexate.

*generic drug—available without prescription upon request to pharmacist

INDEX

KEEP YOURSELF HEALTHY

EARL MINDELL'S VITAMIN BIBLE
Earl Mindell

The author, a certified nutritionist and practicing pharmacist for over fifteen years, has written the most comprehensive and complete book about vitamins and nutrient supplements ever. We learn which vitamin needs vary for each of us and how to determine our individual needs.

Available in paperback (L30-300, $3.75)

THE ALLERGY COOKBOOK AND FOOD-BUYING GUIDE
Pamela Nonken and S. Roger Hirsch, M.D.

One of every ten Americans—more than twenty million of us—suffers from some form of allergy; food allergy is the most difficult to diagnose and treat. This book is a one-of-a-kind book that authoritatively tells you how to completely avoid allergies in planning and cooking meals. A must!

A large format paperback
(L37-173, $6.95, U.S.A.)
(L37-341, $7.95, Canada)